Handbook of
Nursing Procedures

GW00708227

Handbook of Nursing Procedures

Edited by

MARY E. SCHOLES
RGN CMB (Part I) NA Cert (Hosp)
Chief Area Nursing Officer
Tayside Health Board

JANE L. WILSON
BA (Hons) RGN RSCN CMB (Part I)
DN (Part A) RTN MPhil
Director of Nurse Education
Dundee College of Nursing
and Midwifery

SHEILA MACRAE
RGN SCM RCT NA Cert (Hosp)
District Nursing Officer
Dundee District
Tayside Health Board

Blackwell Scientific Publications
OXFORD LONDON EDINBURGH
BOSTON PALO ALTO MELBOURNE

©1982 by
Blackwell Scientific Publications
Editorial offices:
Osney Mead, Oxford OX2 0EL
8 John Street, London WC1N
  2ES
23 Ainslie Place, Edinburgh EH3
  6AJ
52 Beacon Street, Boston
  Massachusetts 02108 USA
667 Lytton Avenue, Palo Alto,
  California 94301, USA
107 Barry Street, Carlton
  Victoria 3053 Austrlia

First published 1982
Reprinted 1983, 1986

Printed and bound in
Great Britain by
Butler & Tanner Ltd
Frome and London

DISTRIBUTORS

USA
  Blackwell Mosby Book
    Distributors
  11830 Westline Industrial Drive
  St Louis, Missouri 63141

Canada
  The C.V. Mosby Company
  5240 Finch Avenue East,
  Scarborough, Ontario

Australia
  Blackwell Scientific Publications
    (Australia) Pty Ltd
  107 Barry Street
  Carlton, Victoria 3053

British Library
Cataloguing in Publication Data

Handbook of nursing procedures.
  1. Nursing
  I. Scholes, Mary E.
  II. Wilson, Jane L.
  III. Macrae, Sheila
  610.73   RT41

ISBN 0–632–00687–0

Contents

List of Figures

Foreword

The difficulty of establishing a uniform pattern of nursing procedures acceptable to all wards and departments within a hospital is too well known to need elaboration. With the move to group schools of nursing in recent years this difficulty has been accentuated.

Dundee College of Nursing, one of the first such colleges to be established, was opened in 1969 to amalgamate all nurse training schools in the Dundee district and had the responsibility to provide programmes of training for the different forms of registration and for enrolment. This presented an even greater need to standardise procedures in classroom and clinical areas and resulted in the setting up of a procedure committee representative of service and teaching staffs. The committee subsequently produced guidelines for the common nursing procedures.

In 1972 Dundee introduced the first comprehensive nurse training programme in Scotland. The programme required every student nurse to be given theory and practical experience relative to the four disciplines for which registration was available and included the community and midwifery fields. It, therefore, became necessary to give further consideration to the teaching of basic nursing procedures.

A short time after the introduction of comprehensive training, Dundee incorporated midwifery training into the work of the college, thus creating Dundee College of Nursing and Midwifery.

In order to meet all these changes the procedure committee was re-convened and enlarged to represent all fields of training used by learners, and in this respect it is worth remembering that training for the Roll in Scotland has been of a multi-discipline nature since 1972.

Those who have been involved in procedure committee work will be only too well aware of the problems faced in endeavouring to reach agreement on matters which the majority of trained nurses have strong personal views. It is a measure of the success of the committee that this handbook has been produced, and it is indeed a credit to all concerned.

The book is issued to all nurse learners and to staff in all areas of training. It has proved very worthwhile, and is an important aid to nurse training.

It is a pleasure to acknowledge the excellent and continuing work of the committee and the ready support of the staff of the Dundee District and the Chief Area Nursing Officer who by their cooperation, have made this publication possible.

F. Ellis   MBE RGN DN RNT
Formerly Director of Nurse Education
Dundee College of Nursing and Midwifery
June 1981

1
Basic Nursing Procedures

*Indicates that Paediatric nursing notes are included

1.1
Bedmaking

Bedmaking is carried out to enhance the patient's comfort, ensure good body alignment and positioning in relation to the patient's condition. During bedmaking it is important to ensure the safety of the patient by applying the bed brakes and to observe the condition of patient and equipment. The nurse will also make beds in such a way as to prevent the spread of infection and development of pressure sores.

Principles
Where possible two people should make a bed working in harmony.

Warmth and privacy must be ensured for the patient.

Handle the patient gently, give support and explain all moves.

Include the patient in any conversation.

If allowed, sit the patient well supported in a chair while the bed is being made.

Change patient's position and carry out skin care if necessary (see Procedure 1.12).

Prevention of infection
Avoid shaking bed clothes.

Keep bed clothes and any other bed aids off the floor.

Discard used or soiled bed clothes immediately into appropriate linen carrier/s.

Observations
Check patient's general condition.
Check any apparatus in use.

1.2
Ordinary occupied bed

Preparation of the patient
Explain the procedure to the patient, note any apparatus or bed equipment in use and patient's position. Ensure that immediate environment is warm, closing nearby windows if necessary.

Equipment
Trolley with clean linen
Carrier/s for used or soiled linen
Bed stripper or two chairs
If required: equipment for *skin care* and/or equipment for *bed bathing* (soiled patient)

Procedure
1   Ensure privacy for the patient.
2   Place bed stripper or two chairs at bottom of the bed.
3   Loosen bed clothes all round, working methodically from top to bottom of bed.
4   Fold off upper bed clothes singly, folding each into three in concertina fashion as far as blanket nearest to patient.
5   Slip out upper sheet in a similar manner leaving the patient covered with a blanket.
6   Remove any bed aids and place on a chair preventing them or the bed clothes removed from touching the floor.
7   Deal with linen under the patient either by the *Rolling* or *Sitting method.*
    Rolling method—for changing or straightening underlinen. One nurse assists or rolls the patient to

one side of the bed supporting him safely in this position, while the other nurse attends to the bed linen. Starting from top to bottom the underlinen is untucked. The undersheet is straightened and any crumbs removed. The side of the undersheet is then tucked in top to bottom with mitred corners. Draw and waterproof sheets are straightened and tucked in. The patient is now assisted or carefully rolled to the other side of the bed and the second nurse repeats the same procedure.

If draw sheet is soiled, remove and replace. If undersheet is soiled, assist or roll the patient to one side of the bed and roll all underlinen closely up to the patient's back. Place clean underlinen, undersheet, draw and waterproof sheets on the unoccupied half of the bed and secure. Assist or roll the patient carefully on to the clean underlinen, undo the roll of clean linen and straighten and tuck in as before.

Sitting method—for changing or straightening underlinen. Assist the patient to move and sit partly down the bed. If patient is unable to do so lift carefully down the bed with the assistance of another nurse (a third nurse may be necessary for an extremely ill or heavy patient). Support the patient in this position using pillows for the patient's comfort as required.

The underlinen is untucked. The undersheet is straightened and any crumbs removed. The sides of undersheet are then tucked in at the top of the bed with mitred corners. Draw and waterproof sheets are straightened and tucked in. Place backrest and pillows in position and assist or carefully lift the patient back up the bed. Repeat the procedure at the bottom of the bed.

Soiled underlinen is changed by placing top half

of undersheet, draw and waterproof sheets on unoccupied top half of the bed, tucking in top parts
and making the remainder into a roll to roll beneath
the patient. The bottom half of the bed is then
tucked in as before.

NOTES. **Always** ensure that the undersheets are
taut.

Pressure area care is given during the stage of attending to underlinen. Also *passive* or *active leg
exercises* and observation of state of lower limbs and
correct limb alignment.

8 Discard used or soiled linen into appropriate
carrier.

9 Replace any bed aids.

10 Put on top sheet, leaving a turnover of about
50 cm at top. Make a pleat at either side at the lower
end of sheet and tuck in all round at foot and sides.
Mitre corners at foot of the bed.

NOTE. **Do not** turn back the sheet at the foot of
the bed unless asked to do so for a *special examination*.

11 Put on blankets, one by one, pleat at the bottom
as for top sheet before tucking in. **Make sure**
the patient's chest is adequately covered. Fold in a
small portion of the corners of the blankets at the
top.

12 Put on bed cover (counterpane) tucking in
lower end only with half mitred corners, fold the
50 cm of top sheet over the bed cover at the top.

NOTES. Again ensure that the patient is comfortable and offer any additional help, e.g. drink,
newspaper. Ensure access to bedside locker.

Ensure safety of the patient by applying bed brake
and securing cot sides (if in use). A variable height
bed may require lowering to meet the patient's requirements.

Paediatric nursing notes

1 When making an occupied cot the sides **must never** be left down—even momentarily—unless a second nurse is present.

2 Linen may be stripped on to cot ends according to ward practice.

3 Heavy duty polythene is used for waterproof sheeting in paediatric wards for toddlers. Older children do not require this unless they are enuretic.

4 Pillows are **not recommended** for children under 1 year of age unless the pillow is placed underneath the mattress.

5 Very few children cannot be lifted out of bed for bedmaking.

6 It is important to **lock cot sides in position** before leaving.

7 Always leave a child with toys or books suitable for his/her stage of development.

1.3
Bedmaking (special beds) — admission

An admission bed is made in a way that facilitates admission of the acutely ill patient and allows bathing of the patient with as little disturbance as possible.

Extra equipment
One long polythene sheet
Two blankets
Any extra apparatus required

Procedure
1 Make up bed as for basic hospital bed as far as the draw sheet.
2 Place one pillow in position then put waterproof sheet and two bath blankets on top.
3 Put top bed clothes on singly, turning up each separately at the bottom.
4 Fold the top bed clothes into a neat pack.

1.4
Bedmaking (special beds) — operation

An operation bed is made in a way which will facilitate easy transfer of the patient from theatre trolley to bed and to have all apparatus required for the patient at the bedside.

Equipment
Clean bed linen
Protective covering for top of the bed, e.g. disposable towel
Any apparatus required for the patient
Appropriate linen carrier

Procedure
1 Make up bed as for basic hospital bed with clean linen as far as the draw sheet.
2 Place protective covering at top of the bed.
3 Put top bed clothes on singly, turning up each separately at the bottom.
4 Fold the top bed clothes into a neat pack.

Paediatric nursing notes
Make up bed with clean linen as far as the draw sheet. Place two sheets on the bed singly, turning up each separately at the bottom. Make up bed.

1.5
Bedmaking (special beds) — orthopaedic

An orthopaedic bed is made to provide a firm base which will support fractures and maintain normal spinal curves.

Extra equipment
Fracture boards (unless bed has a firm base)
Sectional mattress, if available
Bed cage (cradle) and bed elevator if there is a leg injury
Protected pillow if plaster of Paris has been applied

Procedure
1 Place fracture boards under the mattress.
2 Make up bed as for basic hospital bed as far as the draw sheet or place separate sheets on the separate sections (sectional mattress).
3 Place protected pillow in position with bed cage (cradle) on top if plaster of Paris has been applied.
4 Put top bed clothes on singly, turning up each separately at the bottom.
5 Fold top bed clothes into a neat pack.
  NOTES. Bed is left open at the bottom in *leg injuries*.
If balanced traction is used bed clothes are **not tucked in** at the sides of the bed. When a bed cage (cradle) is used a sheet is always placed next to the patient.

1.6
Bedmaking (special beds)—
to relieve dyspnoea or orthopnoea

To relieve dyspnoea or orthopnoea the bed is made to allow the patient to be as comfortable as possible in the upright position.

Extra equipment
Extra pillows and backrest
Foot support and bed cage (cradle)
Bed table and a soft pillow
Covering for the patient's shoulders—bed jacket or
  blanket

Procedure
1   Make up the bed as for basic hospital bed as far as the draw sheet.
2   Pull backrest forward and secure it.
3   Use sufficient pillows to maintain the patient in a comfortable upright position—*dyspnoeic position.*
4   Place foot support and bed cage (cradle) in position and put on top bed clothes in the usual manner. Double folds of blankets **must not** be put over the patient's chest.
5   Provide covering for the patient's shoulders.
6   If the *orthopnoeic position* is preferred by the patient, lift up the bed table with a soft pillow on the table top, once the bed is made, to a position where the patient can comfortably lean forward resting the head and arms on the bed table. To achieve maximum patient comfort it may be necessary to adjust the height of the bed table or bed or both.
    NOTE. Make sure that oxygen is at hand.

1.7
Bedmaking (special beds) —
cots (adult)

Making adult cots varies depending on the type of cot and age of the patient. (See Procedure 1.2.)

   NOTE. It is important to **lock cot sides in position** before leaving the patient.

1.8
Bathing a patient in bed

A patient is bathed in bed in order to cleanse and refresh him/her. The procedure should be explained to the patient and nurse should make sure that the room or immediate area is warm and, if necessary, close nearby windows. The patient's toilet requisites and clean gown/pyjamas should be collected from the locker and he/she should be offered a bedpan/urinal before bathing.

Equipment
Trolley with:
Face cloth ⎫
Body cloth ⎪
Soap in a dish ⎪
Brush and comb ⎬ Collected and usually
Toothbrush and ⎪ available from the
  cleansing agent ⎪ patient's locker
Talcum powder ⎪
Clean gown/pyjamas ⎭
Disposable cloths and towels (for genital areas)
Disposal bag
Nail clippers and scissors in a foil tray
Beaker and mouthwash
Additional equipment for mouth care, as necessary
  (see Procedures 1.13 and 1.14)
Jug of hot water ⎫ **or** ready access to water
Jug of cold water ⎭
Basin and plastic bucket
Bath towel
Face towel

Clean bed linen
Carriers for used or soiled linen
Bed stripper or two chairs

Procedure

1   Take the above equipment to the bedside and ensure privacy for the patient.
2   Place the patient's clean gown/pyjamas, bath towel and face towel to warm on a nearby radiator, if available.
3   Fold off upper bed clothes singly and remove any bed aid/s and place on a chair.
4   Remove as many pillows as possible, depending on the patient's condition and place the patient in a semirecumbent position if comfortable.
5   Remove the patient's gown/pyjamas and encourage the patient to participate in the procedure if able.
6   Expose **only** the part being washed.
7   Wash, rinse and dry each part thoroughly using appropriate towels, paying particular attention to skin folds and powder lightly, if the patient wishes.
8   Adapt the procedure to the patient's needs and condition.
9   Change the water as often as required.
10   If possible place the basin on the bed and allow the patient to wash his/her own face, hands and feet. The patient should be encouraged to attend to his/her own genital hygiene.
11   Attend to the patient's nails if required.

Suggested order of washing
(a) Face, ears and neck.
(b) Arm and hand furthest away from the nurse bathing the patient.
(c) Chest.

(d) Arm and hand nearest to the nùrse bathing the patient.

(e) Abdomen.

(f) Shoulders and back (patient may sit up or roll over). Replace the patient's gown/pyjama jacket or this may be left until the end of the bath.

(g) Change water.

(h) Leg and foot furthest away from the nurse bathing the patient.

(i) Leg and foot nearest to the nurse bathing the patient.

(j) Buttocks and groin.

(k) Genital area— if the patient attends to this he/she should be given the opportunity to wash his/her hands in fresh water on completion of the genital toilet.

12   Replace gown/pyjamas and if the patient is helpless ensure that he/she is placed in an altered position at the end of the procedure.

13   Replace the pillows and bed aid/s and make up the patient's bed with clean linen as necessary.

14   Allow the patient to clean his/her teeth or do this for him/her.

15   Comb or brush the patient's hair or let the patient do so in front of a mirror.

16   Remove bed screens and leave the patient warm and comfortable and offer any additional requirements, e.g. drink, newspaper. Ensure access to the bedside locker.

NOTE. Ensure safety of the patient by applying bed brake and securing cot sides (if in use).

Aftercare of equipment

Place used bath and face towels, bed linen, if necessary, in appropriate laundry container.

Place used disposable cloths and towels in the disposal bag and place in appropriate container.

Clean and wash all equipment including the trolley with detergent and hot water and/or recommended disinfectant.

Wash the patient's toilet requisites and return along with the patient's used personal linen to the patient's locker.

Observation and reporting

Note the conditions of the patient's skin and general appearance and report any abnormality to the nurse in charge.

1.9
Bathing a patient in the bathroom

If at all possible a patient is bathed in the bathroom to cleanse and refresh the patient.

Preparation of the bathroom

Close window/s and place or draw screen between bath and door.

Put 'Engaged' notice on bathroom door.

Position a chair close to the bath and place a disposable bath mat on the floor.

Position antislip mat in the bath (if available).

Place the patient's clean gown/pyjamas, bath towel and face towel on warm towel rail or radiator.

Equipment

Face cloth	
Body cloth	
Soap in a dish	
Brush and comb	Usually available
Toothbrush and	from the patient's
cleansing agent	locker
Talcum powder	
Clean gown/pyjamas	

Disposable cloths and towels (for genital areas)
Disposal bag
Bath thermometer
Disinfectant lotion as recommended
Nail clippers and scissors in a foil tray
Bath towel
Face towel

Preparation of the patient

Enquire from a nurse in charge if the patient can be left alone to bathe.

Explain the procedure to the patient.

Screen bed and assist the patient to put on dressing gown and slippers.

Assist patient to walk to the bathroom or provide conveyance.

If patient has jewellery ensure all the safety precautions are taken.

Procedure

1 Enquire if the patient wishes to go to the toilet before bathing.

2 Let the patient wash face and hands in the washhand basin. The patient may also attend to oral hygiene at this time.

3 While the patient is attending to 2 above, run the bath allowing the cold water to run in first and add the recommended lotion. **Ensure** that the hot and cold water are thoroughly mixed before taking the temperature of the bath water (40°C).

4 Assist the patient to undress, hang up the patient's dressing gown and assist the patient into the bath, if necessary. Neatly fold the patient's used gown/pyjamas in preparation for return to the patient's locker on completion of the bath.

5 If the patient can be left alone to bathe ensure privacy but remain within call. Before leaving instruct the patient in the operation of the nurse-call alarm. (See the following Special nursing notes and Paediatric nursing notes.)

6 If the patient requires assistance to bathe wash and rinse each part in a systematic manner using body or disposable cloths as appropriate. The

patient should be encouraged to attend to his/her own genital hygiene.

7   Assist the patient out of the bath and dry the patient thoroughly using appropriate towels, paying particular attention to skin folds and powder lightly if the patient wishes.

8   Drain the bath and assist the patient to dress.

9   Attend to the patient's nails, if required.

10   Comb or brush the patient's hair or let patient do own in front of a mirror.

11   Assist the patient by the appropriate means back to bed or to sit in a chair in the ward or day room. Leave the patient warm and comfortable and offer any additional requirements, e.g. drink, magazine.

12   If necessary change and remake the patient's bed.

Aftercare of equipment

Return to bathroom and thoroughly clean the bath and wash-hand basin using cleaning agent as recommended.

Wash and hang up antislip mat to dry.

Place used bath and face towels if necessary in appropriate laundry container.

Place used cloths, towels and bath mat in the appropriate containers.

Wash the patient's toilet requisites and return along with the patient's used personal linen to the patient's locker.

Open bathroom window/s. Put 'Vacant' notice on bathroom door and return chair and bathroom screens to their normal position.

Observations and reporting

Note the condition of the patient's skin and general appearance.

Observe the patient's reaction and condition throughout the procedure.

Report any abnormality to the nurse in charge.

NOTE. If the patient becomes dizzy or unfit immediately drain the bath and call for help—**never** leave the patient alone. Note the patient's condition.

Special nursing notes

Certain patients, e.g. potentially suicidal, epileptic, are **never left alone** to bathe even though they are able to bathe themselves. **Always** check with the nurse in charge if the patient can be left alone.

Always obtain help to lift a patient in and out of the bath, or if available use mechanical lift. Explain all moves to the patient.

Always check that moveable equipment, e.g. chair/mechanical lift is secure before lifting or assisting the patient to or from it.

Ensure at all times that the bathroom floor is dry in the interests of nurse and patient safety.

Paediatric nursing notes

Children are usually fully dressed after bathing unless otherwise specified.

Children are **never left alone** in the bathroom at any time.

1.10
Assisting a patient to have a shower

A shower is given to cleanse and refresh the patient.

Preparation of the shower area
See Procedure 1.9, preparation of the bathroom.
Position antislip mat in shower base.
Position a chair close to the shower and place disposable bath mat on floor.

Equipment
As for Procedure 1.9 with the exception of a bath thermometer and the recommended disinfectant lotion.

Plus a shower cap or shampoo if required.
If available, the nurse should wear a protective apron and rubber boots.

Preparation of the patient
As per Procedure 1.9.

Procedure
1   Adjust shower water tap/s to give an even flow of warm water (35–40°C).
2   If necessary assist the patient to undress and to stand under the shower. If unable to stand unsupported push the patient into the shower sitting on a toilet chair.
3   When showering is completed give the same care as for bathing in the bathroom (see Procedure 1.9).

Aftercare of equipment
As per Procedure 1.9.

Observation and reporting
As for Procedure 1.9.

NOTE. **If the patient becomes dizzy** or unfit immediately turn off the shower. If possible **remove the patient** from the shower and sit him/her on the chair. **Call for help—never** leave the patient alone. Note the patient's condition.

Special nursing notes
As for Procedure 1.9.

It is recommended that the nurse should wear protective apron and rubber boots provided during this procedure when appropriate.

1.11
Tepid sponging

Tepid sponging is carried out to reduce a body temperature above 39.4°C by 0.5–1°C.

Equipment
Trolley with:
Bowl of warm water (33°C)
Bowl of ice (for cold compress)
Lotion thermometer
Six cloths or sponges
Face towel and bath towel
Clean bed linen
Clean gown/pyjamas (usually available from the patient's locker)
Carrier/s for used or soiled linen
Bed stripper or two chairs
Additional equipment for mouth care, as necessary (see Procedures 1.13 and 1.14)

Preparation of the patient
Explain the procedure to the patient. Take and record the patient's body temperature (*initial temperature*).
Take trolley to the bedside and screen the bed.
Strip the bed and remove the patient's gown/pyjamas and any bed appliances leaving the patient covered with the top sheet.
Neatly fold the patient's used gown/pyjamas and place in the patient's locker.

Procedure

1 Check the temperature of the bowl of warm water.

2 Gently sponge and pat dry the patient's face and neck.

3 Apply a cold compress to the patient's forehead and change it at intervals during the procedure.

4 Carry out the sponging systematically as for the method suggested in Procedure 1.8—using in this instance long sweeping strokes. Gently pat parts dry, if required.

5 Place wet cloths or sponges in the patient's axillae and groins and renew these as they become warm.

6 Remove cold compresses when attending to the patient's shoulders and back.

7 Change the sheets.

8 Dress the patient in clean gown/pyjamas (synthetic materials, e.g. nylon should be avoided).

9 Remake the bed with clean linen and replace any bed appliances.

10 Attend to the patient's oral hygiene, if required, and leave the patient comfortable. If allowed the patient can be given a cool drink.

11 Unscreen the bed and remove the equipment.

12 30 minutes after completion of the procedure return and take and record the patient's body temperature (*secondary temperature*). Chart this below the patients *initial temperature*, i.e. the temperature which was taken before the procedure commenced.

Aftercare of equipment

Clean and wash trolley and bowls with detergent and hot water or recommended disinfectant.

Place used bath and face towels and bed linen in appropriate laundry container.

Place used cloths or sponges (if disposable) in a disposal bag and place in the appropriate container.

Reporting

Report the patient's body temperatures prior to and after treatment to the nurse in charge.

NOTE. Should the patient start to shiver during any stage of the procedure—**stop immediately** and cover the patient with a blanket and report to the nurse in charge.

Paediatric nursing notes

A child's temperature may be reduced by:

Exposure: remove all clothing with the exception of a terry towelling nappy.

Fanning: if child's body temperature is above 38°C an electric fan is placed on the bedside locker. **Note** the fan must be **out of the reach** of the child and other children in the ward. When fanning, the child's extremities may need to be covered and at **all** times regular temperature checks must be taken and recorded in accordance with medical instructions.

Tepid sponging.

Use of antipyretic drug as prescribed.

1.12
Prevention of pressure sores/decubitus ulcers

A pressure sore, or decubitus ulcer, is a term used to describe a sore on the body resulting from any of the following causes:

1   Pressure. May be from the weight of the patient's body itself. Parts at risk include the back of the head, shoulders, elbows, sacrum, knees, ankles and heels. Pressure may also occur from the weight of bed clothes, from wrinkles in sheets or from plaster of Paris casts or splints or improperly used bed appliances.

2   Shearing force. Dragging of tissues away from the bone. May occur when patient **slips down** the bed or is **pulled up** the bed. The blood supply to the deep tissues is cut off and a deep blue patch can develop over the affected area which may later break down.

3   Friction. Many things cause friction which roughens the patient's skin and makes it easier to break, e.g. crumbs, hard sheet, wrinkles or two skin surfaces rubbing against each other.

4   Moisture. A wet skin, even with plain water will break down more easily than a dry skin, but if the moisture is urine, faeces or discharge the hazard is even greater because of the acid or alkaline content of the substance.

Patients at risk
Patients at risk are those who cannot move easily,

e.g. the elderly or paralysed patients, and those who are emaciated.

Prevention

1 Relieve pressure. Can be achieved by early ambulation where this is possible. If not, regular changing of position, regular patient exercises— *passive* or *active*—will help. When the patient's position cannot be changed regularly aids to relieve or reduce pressure may be used, e.g. ripple mattresses, sheepskins, tubipads, bed cages (cradles) bedrings, etc. Nurses are reminded of the importance of having bottom sheets kept taut.

2 Shearing force. Prevented by placing a support at the patient's feet to prevent him/her slipping down the bed and by lifting the patient **clear** of the mattress when moving him/her up or down the bed or to and from the bed.

3 Friction. A smooth, crumb free bed and gown/pyjamas will help to reduce and prevent friction.

4 Moisture. Regular washing, rinsing and drying of the patient's skin; changing of patient's clothing whenever it becomes wet or soiled from whatever reason will do a great deal to reduce or prevent sores caused by moisture. The application of a lubricant cream may be necessary when hygiene is complete.

5 The patient should have an adequate diet.

6 Jewellery, e.g. dress ring and wrist watches which could accidentally damage the patient's skin **must not** be worn by any nursing staff.

7 Nursing staff should keep fingernails short and neat and skin smooth.

NOTE. If a pressure sore occurs it **must be treated** as a surgical dressing (see Procedures 3.17 and 3.18).

1.13
Regular mouth care

In health the mouth is kept clean by:
  a normal diet containing plenty of fresh foods and
    fluids
  the flow of saliva—which is encouraged by the
    use of lemon or lime drinks
  regular cleaning of teeth
The aims of oral hygiene procedures are to:
  afford the patient a fresh tasting mouth and a
    fresh breath and to enhance the enjoyment of
    food
  prevent tooth decay, a coated tongue, cracked lips
    and sores, e.g. oral ulcers
  prevent complications arising from the spread of
    infection, e.g. parotitis

Preparation of the patient
Explain the procedure to the patient and help the
patient sit up in a comfortable position, if allowed.

Equipment
Tray with:
Toothbrush and cleansing agent (each patient
  should have his/her own)
Denture bowl or box (labelled with the patient's
  name), if required
A mouthwash in a tumbler or disposable mug, e.g.
  glycerine of thymol 25% solution or mouthwash
  tablets
Bowl for return of mouthwash and water
Glass of water

Disposable tissues
Disposal bag

Procedure
1   Ensure privacy for the patient.
2   Assist the patient, if necessary, to clean his/her teeth and rinse out his/her mouth. Ask the patient to remove his/her denture/s and place them in the denture bowl or box. (If the patient is unable to do this use a disposable tissue and remove the patient's denture/s.)
3   Take the patient's denture/s in the denture bowl or box to the bathroom and thoroughly clean them with toothbrush and cleansing agent (paste or powder). Rinse the dentures on completion of cleaning.
4   Return the denture/s to the patient in clean cold water.
5   Assist the patient, if necessary, to have a mouthwash.
6   Ask the patient to replace the denture/s. (If the patient is unable to do this use a disposable tissue and replace the denture/s.)
7   Pour the patient a drink, if required.
8   Leave the patient comfortable.
9   Unscreen the bed and remove the equipment.

Aftercare of equipment
Wash and clean all equipment with detergent and hot water or recommended disinfectant.
Wash the patient's toothbrush and return it along with the patient's tooth paste/powder to the patient's locker.
Place disposable bag containing the used disposable tissues and the disposable mug (if used) into the appropriate container.

Observation and reporting

Note the condition of the patient's mouth, tongue, lips and gums and report any abnormalities to the nurse in charge.

Paediatric nursing notes

1   Children's teeth are cleaned after meals and last thing at night.

2   Some conditions, **e.g.** stomatitis may require the application of gentian violet 1% in aqueous solution. Strict attention should be paid to crockery and cutlery in such cases.

3   Cleaning the mouth of a child should only be required if the child is unconscious or too debilitated to have teeth cleaned (see Procedure 1.14).

1.14
Cleaning the mouth of a helpless patient

When a patient is unconscious or acutely ill **special mouth care must** be given at frequent intervals, e.g. hourly or 2 hourly. Individual equipment **must** be used—each patient should have a tray set for his/her own requirements. Disposable equipment is used whenever possible. The nurse **must** wash his/her hands carefully before and after each treatment.

Preparation of the conscious patient
Explain the procedure to the patient and help the patient to sit up in a comfortable position, supported by pillows, if allowed.

Equipment
A tray is set with:
A disposable dressing towel
Disposable tissues
Gauze swabs
Wooden or plastic tongue depressor
1 gallipot or small foil bowl containing sodium bicarbonate 0.625% solution
1 gallipot or small foil bowl containing glycerine of thymol 25% solution
1 pair swab-holding forceps (artery forceps)
1 pair dissecting forceps
Soft white paraffin
Denture bowl or box (labelled with the patient's name)

Toothbrush and cleansing agent (each patient
  should have his/her own)
Mouthwash and receiver if patient is conscious
Disposal bag
A good light

Procedure
1   Ensure privacy for the patient.
2   Place the dressing towel under the patient's chin
and remove the denture/s, if any, using a disposable
tissue and place them in the denture bowl or box.
3   Examine the patient's mouth thoroughly in a
good light. Note the condition of the tongue and
lips and the presence of sores or ulceration.
4   Place gauze swab in swab-holding forceps, dip
in sodium bicarbonate solution and moisten the lips
and clean the vestibule of the patient's mouth (including the cheeks and the gums at one side of the
mouth). Remove the swab from the swab-holding
forceps, using the dissecting forceps and place the
used swab in the disposal bag.
   NOTE. In certain case the nurse in charge can be
consulted about using a gloved finger.
5   Repeat the procedure (item 4) for the other side
of the patient's mouth.
6   Clean the cavity of the patient's mouth, including gums, teeth, roof of the mouth and the tongue
using a clean swab for each part. Clean the tongue
from side to side.
7   The patient may then, if conscious or able to do
so have a mouthwash.
8   **If the patient is unconscious** repeat the whole
procedure (items 4, 5 and 6) using glycerine of thymol, then smear the patient's lips with soft white
paraffin.
9   Take the patient's denture/s in the denture bowl

or box to the bathroom and thoroughly clean and return as per Procedure 1.13.

10   Continue procedure as per items 6, 7, 8 and 9 of Procedure 1.13.

Aftercare equipment
As per Procedure 1.13.

Observation and reporting
As per Procedure 1.13.

1.15
General care of the hair

It is necessary to keep the patient's hair in good condition and to make the patient feel more comfortable and boost his/her morale.

Equipment
Each patient should have his/her own brush and/or comb and also a hand mirror.

Procedure
1   Brush and/or comb the patient's hair, doing matted hair strand by strand.
2   Leave the patient's hair in its normal style. Use hand mirror to show the patient.
3   If time permits, the nurse may help the female patient to set her hair.
4   The patient's hair should be washed regularly, and brushed and/or combed at least twice daily.

Aftercare of equipment
The patient's brush and/or comb should be washed and cleaned regularly.

Observation and reporting
Note the condition of patient's scalp and hair and report any abnormalities to the nurse in charge.

Special nursing note
Before and after an electro-encephalogram (EEG) a patient's hair is thoroughly washed.

1.16
Hair inspection

Hair inspection facilitates early cleansing of a verminous head and prevents the spread of infestation.
Adults: Inspect hair on admission, as directed and
on discharge.
Children: All children have their hair inspected on
admission and daily thereafter and the condition of
same is recorded.

Preparation of the patient
Tray with:
Large disposable towel
Dressing and fine tooth combs in a foil tray
Cotton wool mops
Gallipot or small foil bowl of antiseptic, e.g. Savlon
   1% solution
Disposal bag
Mirror

Procedure
1   Ensure privacy for the patient.
2   Fix the disposable towel around the patient's
shoulders.
3   Remove all the patient's hair grips.
4   Part the patient's hair with the dressing comb.
5   Using a fine tooth comb, comb the patient's hair
strand by strand, holding a damp cotton wool mop
under the comb to trap any pediculi and wipe the
comb.
6   Examine the comb and the wool mop.
7   Examine the patient's hair carefully for the pres-

ence of nits, particularly behind the ears and the nape of the neck and note the condition of the scalp.

8   Leave the patient's hair in its normal style—use the mirror to show the patient.

9   Leave the patient warm and comfortable.

10   Unscreen the bed and remove the tray.

Aftercare of equipment

Scrub and wash all the combs in the recommended lotion then rinse and dry.

Place disposal bag containing used disposable equipment in the appropriate container.

Return the patient's comb to the bedside locker.

Reporting

Report and record the condition of the patient's hair and scalp to the nurse in charge and if the patient's head is verminous carry out the prescribed treatment at once (see Procedure 1.17).

1.17
Treatment of a verminous head

Verminous head treatment is carried out to apply a substance which will destroy pediculi and that will also kill the nits as they hatch out; and to promote health, to improve the patient's comfort and prevent the spread of infestation.

Preparation of the patient
Explain the procedure tactfully to the patient and assist the patient into a sitting-up position, if possible.

Equipment
Tray with:
Large disposable towels
Dressing comb in a foil tray
Cotton wool mops
Disposal bag
Prescribed vermicide
Gallipot or small foil bowl for emulsion (if used)
Disposable gown, cap and gloves

Procedure
1   Ensure privacy for the patient.
2   Nurse dons disposable gown, cap and gloves.
3   Arrange disposable towels around the patient's shoulders.
4   Remove all the patient's hair grips and part the patient's hair with the dressing comb.

5 Read and carry out the directions on the container of whichever vermicide is used, taking care to ensure that the whole of the patient's scalp is treated.

6 Leave the patient's hair tidy and remove the disposable towel and place in disposal bag.

7 Remove the disposable gown, cap and gloves and place in disposal bag.

8 Leave the patient comfortable.

9 Unscreen the bed and remove the tray.

Aftercare of equipment
As per Procedure 1.16.

Aftercare of the patient
Wash the patient's hair 24 hours after the treatment. Repeat the treatment if necessary.

Observations and reporting
Report to the nurse in charge:

1 The patient's reaction to the condition and to the treatment.

2 The extent of the infestation and the condition of the patient's scalp. Record the treatment in a special book and report the condition daily.

   NOTE. Some pediculi are resistant to certain vermicides.

Paediatric nursing notes
It is important to inform the parent/s of the state of the child's head on admission.
Acetic acid 1% solution is used to loosen nits.

1.18
Toilet facilities

The provision of toilet facilities is particularly important for the following reasons:

Patient's comfort. The **maximum** amount of privacy should be afforded to the patient at all times as well as the **minimum** of incurred inconvenience.

Patient safety. The maximum patient safety is achieved by ensuring that the brake/s on sanichairs and commodes are in the locked position when in use and by ensuring the nurse-call alarm or bell is within the patient's reach.

Prevention of infection. Urine and faeces contain infective material and care **must** be taken to prevent the spread of infection. Bed patient's **must** be provided with handwashing facilities. Nurses **must** wash their hands carefully after each procedure.

Observation of excreta. All patient excreta must be observed before disposal and any abnormality reported to the nurse in charge. Abnormal excreta must be kept for inspection.

Specimens should be prepared as requested.

The measuring and recording of urinary output **must** be carried out accurately.

Types of toilet equipment in common use

Bedpan: used much less now, but still the only method of value in many instances. It may be made of stainless steel, polythene or plastic, the latter is used with a disposable compressed paper composite lining or insert.

Urinal: type of bottle made from the same materials as a bedpan and is commonly used for urination by the non-ambulant male patient. Special urinals are also available for the non-ambulant female patient.

Commode chair: chair with a toilet bowl which may be wheeled to the patient's bedside. The patient is lifted or assisted out of bed on to the commode so that a more natural position is provided.

Sanichair: a portable lavatory-type chair on which the patient can be taken to the lavatory.

Giving toilet equipment

In all wards and departments toilet facilities are available, as and when required. In some instances the ward is closed to visitors at regular times and a *toilet round* is carried out, using various toilet equipment but observing individual patient privacy. A special heated trolley is used to transport clean bedpans. Used bedpans are collected singly after use on a separate collecting trolley. Handwashing facilities **must** always be made available for each patient.

Observations and reporting

Note and report any discomfort or pain the patient may have when passing urine or faeces.

Inspect contents of utensil before disposal and report same.

Measure and chart urinary output **immediately** if a fluid balance chart is being used for the patient.

Collect and label specimens as required.

NOTE. Nursing staff **must** adhere to the rules for handwashing.

1.19
Giving a bedpan

Preparation of the patient
Explain each step of the procedure to the patient and gain his/her cooperation.
Encourage independence.

Equipment
Trolley with:
Warm bedpan or a bedpan plastic former with a disposable compressed composite paper insert covered with disposable paper bedpan cover
Covered urinal for male patient
Toilet tissues or paper
Disposable cloths and towel (for perineal area)
Disposable hand towel/s
Bowl of warm water (33–35°C) for washing perineal area
Basin of warm water (33–35°C) for patient hand-washing
Disposal bag
Clean bed linen, if necessary

Procedure
1   Ensure complete privacy for the patient and help him/her to relax.
2   Loosen top bed clothes and fold them back without exposing the patient.
3   Suitably arrange the patient's bedwear and place the bedpan on the edge of the bed.
4   Affording adequate support lift the patient's buttocks clear of the bed and slip the bedpan under

him/her to an appropriate position in the centre of the bed. Ensure that the patient is adequately supported and comfortable, if possible, but staying within call in case help is needed. **Never** leave the patient sitting on a bedpan longer than is necessary.

5   When toilet is complete, roll the patient gently over on to his/her side and carefully remove the bedpan. The bedpan is then covered and placed on the trolley.

6   Clean the patient with toilet tissues or paper and place these in the disposal bag.

7   Wash and dry the perineal area.

8   Straighten and tighten all bottom bed linen.

9   Position patient comfortably and remake patient's bed with clean linen, if required.

10   Allow patient to wash his/her hands.

11   Unscreen the bed and open nearby window, use deodorant (air-freshener) if necessary. Remove the trolley.

Aftercare of equipment
Attend to the contents of the bedpan in the sluice and note any abnormality. Retain abnormal excreta for inspection.

With disposable forceps, remove dressings of cotton wool which may be present in the bedpan. **Do not put these down the drain** but place in the appropriate container. A stainless steel bedpan is flushed and cleaned and placed in the steriliser. Disposable bedpan paper insert is discarded into appropriate unit to be pulverised and the plastic bedpan former is washed and cleaned with detergent and hot water and/or recommended disinfectant.

Any additional equipment used in the sluice, e.g. measuring jug is washed and cleaned after use.

Wash the outside of collection bottle, if in use.
NOTE. Wash hands **thoroughly.**

Observation and reporting
As per Procedure 1.17.

Nursing note
For a bowel movement the male patient is given
both a bedpan and a urinal.

1.20
Giving a urinal

Preparation of the patient
As per Procedure 1.19.

Equipment
Urinal
Urinal cover
Bowl of warm water (33–35°C) for patient handwashing
Disposable hand towel/s
Disposal bag

Procedure
1   Ensure complete privacy for the patient.
2   Loosen top bed clothes and fold them back without exposing the patient.
3   Give patient the urinal which is collected **immediately** after use. Helpless patient will, however, require assistance.
4   Straighten and tighten all bottom bed linen.
5   Position the patient comfortably and remake the patient's bed using clean linen, if required.
6   Allow the patient to wash his hands.
7   Unscreen the bed and remove equipment.

Aftercare of equipment
As per Procedure 1.19.

Observation and reporting
As per Procedure 1.18.

1.21
Giving a commode

Preparation of the patient
As per Procedure 1.19.

Equipment
As per Procedure 1.19 with the exception of covered
bedpan and covered urinal for the male patient **plus**
a commode.

Procedure
1   Take commode plus trolley to patient's bedside.
2   Ensure complete privacy for the patient.
3   Check that both bed and commode brakes are in
the locked (ON) position.
4   Fold back the bed clothes and assist the patient
to sit supported over the edge of the bed. Put on the
patient's socks and slippers.
5   With assistance help the patient to stand on the
floor, taking care to ensure that his/her feet do not
slip on the floor. While the patient is being assisted
to stand, free the patient's bedwear from his/her
buttocks. Gently lower the patient to sit on the
commode.
6   Put the patient's arms into his/her dressing
gown in an appropriate way. The patient should be
kept warm.
7   Stay within call.
8   When toilet is complete, provide the necessary
toilet hygiene and handwashing facilities for the
patient.
9   Remove the patient's dressing gown, fold neatly

and place in the patient's locker, and with assistance help or lift the patient back to bed which has been made comfortable during his/her absence. While the patient is being assisted back to bed pull up/down the patient's bedwear.

10 Remove the patient's socks and slippers and place them in the bedside locker. Ensure that the patient is comfortable.

11 Unscreen the bed and open nearby window, use deodorant (air-freshener) if necessary. Remove commode and trolley.

Aftercare of equipment
As per Procedure 1.19 plus washing of commode seat.

Observation and reporting
As per Procedure 1.18.

1.22
Giving a sanichair

The procedure for giving a sanichair is similar to
that of giving a commode (see Procedure 1.21) but
the nurse takes the patient to the lavatory.

Preparation of the patient
Explain the procedure to the patient and with assistance, if required, help the patient up out of bed and
dress in his/her dressing gown, socks and slippers.
Transport the patient in the sanichair to the lavatory.

Procedure in lavatory
1   Raise lavatory seat and carefully wheel the sanichair in reverse over the toilet pan.
2   Apply brake/s on the chair.
3   Free the patient's bedwear from his/her buttocks and ensure that the patient is comfortable.
4   Stay within call to afford any assistance required.
5   When toilet is complete observe contents of the
toilet pan before flushing.
6   Allow the patient to use the washhand basin.
7   Then return the patient to his/her bed, remove
his/her dressing gown, fold it neatly and place in
the patient's locker.
8   With assistance, if required, help the patient
back to bed and remove his/her socks and slippers
and place them in the bedside locker.
9   Leave the patient warm and comfortable and
remove the sanichair.

Aftercare of equipment

As per Procedure 1.19 plus washing of sanichair seat.

Observation and reporting

As per Procedure 1.18.

Special care of the female patient. Special facilities for washing and changing should be made available for female bed patients during menstruation.

Many female patients prefer to use the Bidet for post elimination hygiene. A bidet is a type of open toilet with a warm water spray, foot or hand controlled, used for irrigation after toilet.

Paediatric nursing notes

Toilet training in toddlers. Toddlers should be placed on a potty after every meal and praised if they have performed.

1.23
Last offices

The immediate hospital care after confirmation of death by a doctor that a patient has died is called the last offices.

It is **important to note** the following points:

Verification of the death in hospital should always be the responsibility of a doctor.

In all hospitals, when a patient is believed to have died and a doctor is not present at the time, the normal procedure should be for the nursing staff to notify the doctor on duty and for the doctor to attend, as soon as possible to verify death. The body should not be removed from the ward, nor the relatives notified of the death until this has been done.

If a patient is considered in imminent danger of death this should be recorded and the relatives informed by the nurse in charge.

In all cases where the Procurator Fiscal or Coroner requires to be notified endotracheal tubes, intravenous giving sets, etc. should be left as they are, whether the death occurs in theatre areas or in the wards or in any other part of Health Service premises, subject, of course, to moving the body to a suitable location.

Procedure following confirmation of death

1   The persons who must be notified immediately after medical confirmation of death are:

the parents or the relatives of the patient

the nursing officer or deputy

the house physician/surgeon if the on-call doctor

has certified death. The house physician surgeon will notify the patient's general practitioner

2   In the case of sudden death of a Roman Catholic patient who has not received the Last Rites, the priest must be notified.

If a member of a particular religious denomination is needed in the event of expected or sudden death, the hospital switchboard telephonist normally has a list of available ministers.

3   Official Notices of Death are made out and distributed to the following:

the Nursing Administration with day/night report

the head porter

the records office with the daily returns

NOTE. The procedure following confirmation of death may vary in individual hospitals.

Primary part of last offices
When death has been confirmed carry out the primary part of the last offices procedure.

1   Ensure that the curtains or screen are drawn closely around the bed. A child, if possible, should be in a side room.

2   Remove the top bed clothes leaving a sheet to cover the patient.

3   Lay the patient flat with one pillow.

4   Gently close the patient's eyes and, if necessary, place moist cotton wool swabs on the patient's eyelids.

5   Clean the patient's mouth and replace any dentures.

6   Support the patient's jaw with a light pillow or by a light bandage.

7 Place the patient's limbs in a natural position with the arms by the sides.

8 Leave the patient covered by a sheet.

NOTE. There is usually no need to carry out the final part of the last offices procedure at once. The body can be left for 1 hour, unless the relatives are waiting or expected.

Final part of last offices
Equipment
Prepare a bed-bathing trolley (see Procedure 1.8) excluding clean gown/pyjamas, beaker and mouth-wash plus:

Dressing pack
Cotton wool balls
Waterproof strapping
Disposable forceps
Disposable scissors
Shaving equipment
Disposal bags
Protective gown or apron for nursing staff
Safety pins for pinning mortuary sheet
Shroud
Mortuary sheet and identification labels

Procedure
1 Remove all tubes except endotracheal tubes, re-dress any wound and cover with waterproof strapping to prevent leakage except in deaths where the Procurator Fiscal or Coroner must be informed.

2 Wash the patient.

3 Lightly plug the rectal orifice with cotton wool using disposable forceps. If necessary plug other orifices. In the case of a small child apply a dispos-able napkin with a polythene backing.

4   A label with the patient's name and relevant details should be tied to the patient's big toe. In the case of a small baby the label is tied to the ankles. The ankles and also the knees should be tied together. In certain cases this procedure varies and nurse in charge should be consulted.

5   Place the shroud in position. A small infant is dressed.

NOTE. In the case of children, if parent/s are not present at death and wish to see their child it is often kinder to allow them to do so in the ward where the child may be dressed in clothes. The child's hands may be clasped and fingers entwined with a small flower placed in the hands.

6   Wrap the body in the mortuary sheet using pins to secure the sheet. A small infant is wrapped in a small mortuary wrap.

7   A label, giving details of the patient is attached either to the front of the shroud or mortuary sheet or wrap.

8   Inform the head porter's office that the body is ready for removal. State age of a child.

9   The patient's property is collected and listed and a second nurse **must** check these items. Any valuables are locked up in the appropriate place. Soiled articles of clothing should be placed in a separate bag. All of the patient's personal property must be clearly labelled.

10   The relatives must sign a receipt on receiving the deceased patient's articles.

Aftercare of equipment
As per Procedure 1.8

Special nursing notes
In the community the procedure of last offices is normally carried out by an undertaker.

All of the patient's jewellery should be removed unless otherwise instructed by a relative. This should be noted in the receipt for the patient's articles.

2
Lifting Procedures

2.1
Techniques for lifting patients

Lifting occupies a great deal of a nurse's time and energy. Every nursing situation which includes lifting is different and for each the nurse must select a lift which will cause the least discomfort to the patient. In the majority of lifting situations assistance should be obtained and the nurse should direct such assistance in the use of correct lifting techniques. This is important not only for the patient's safety and comfort but also for the nurse and her/his assistant/s.

Principles in lifting
The main principles in lifting (see Fig. 1) are:

Lift with a **straight back** to protect ligaments, muscles and joints.

Lift with **head erect** and **chin tucked in** to help keep back straight.

Lift with **knees bent** to control buttocks and thigh muscles.

Lift with **feet apart** (approximately hip width) to give a stable base and to allow for a good transference of weight.

Lift with **elbows close to sides** to utilise muscle force efficiently. When lifting with assistance **ensure firm hand grip/s** or wrist grip/s.

Rules for lifting
Always **assess the lifting situation** and always try to obtain assistance, even in an emergency situation.

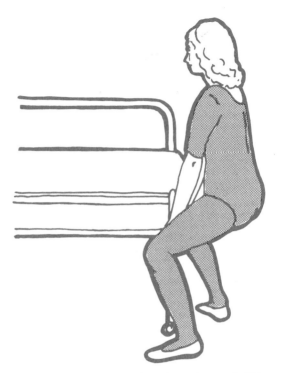

Fig. 1 The main principles of position and stance in lifting.

Always **select a suitable lift** and agree the method
of lifting with the assistant and decide who will
lead the lifting procedure and the signal to commence the lift.

Always **explain the lift to the patient** and explain
how he/she can assist.

Always **remove any items of ward furniture**
from lifting area to give the lifters a clear lifting
pathway.

Always **test the weight** before lifting and if too
heavy obtain further assistance.

Always **signal the moment to lift** so that the lifters and the patient can move together.

Always after completion of the lift make sure the patient is comfortable and replace any items of ward furniture.

Predisposing factors to injury
Injury may be sustained while lifting for the following reasons:

Faulty lifting technique.

Lifting too heavy a weight.

Sudden lifting, causing sudden strain. Always prepare for lifting and avoid tension.

Lifting with turning and twisting at the same time. During a lift the body **must** always be poised with good muscle balance. Adjustment of balance between the upward lift and the turn must take place independently.

Lifters of noticeable unequal height and build throwing additional strain on one lifter.

Heavy lifting on a slippery surface. The floor should be dry and non-skid as should the sides of footwear.

Mechanical lifting machines
Mechanical lifting machines must be used according to the makers instructions and in situations for which they were specifically designed.

Types of lifts in common use
Shoulder or Australian lift

Orthodox or traditional (cradle) lift

Stretcher or trolley lift

These three lifts are described in detail on the following pages.

2

Community nursing service

Modified lifting procedures are used in nursing and care situations in the community. Figure 2 shows a nurse assisting a patient to stand, and (Fig. 2c) supporting or steadying the standing patient.

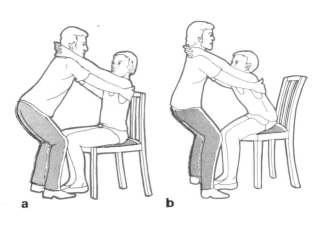

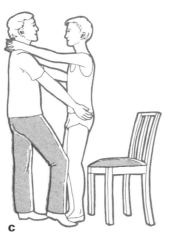

Fig. 2 Assisting a patient (a and b) to stand (c), using a modified lifting procedure.

2.2
Shoulder or Australian lift
(2 lifters)

Common uses
Moving the patient up the bed.
Moving the patient from bed to chair.

Special nursing note
The shoulder or Australian lift is **never** used for
the hemiplegic patient **or** where the patient has a
painful shoulder or axilla.

Shoulder lift up the bed
Position of the patient. Sitting with legs extended
or flexed with arms resting easily over the nurses'
backs (Fig. 3a).
Position of the lifters. Facing the head of the bed
with the shoulders square (Fig. 3b). The leading
foot of each lifter pointing in the direction of movement. The lifters should stand as close in to the
patient as possible. The lifters' hips and knees are
flexed just sufficiently to position their shoulders
accurately in relation to the patient's axilla. The **tip
of the near** shoulder goes into the patient's axilla.
Grasp. The arm nearest the patient is used to
grasp under the patient's thighs. The free hand is
placed firmly on the bed behind the patient's back
to help push up.
NOTE. The two lifters **must** get their shoulders
level and well into the patient's axillae.
The lift. To the command **'Ready' — 'Lift'** the
hips and knees are extended and the shoulder girdle
muscles lift the patient **up** off the bed and by means

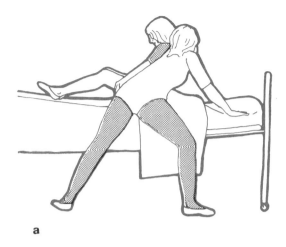

a

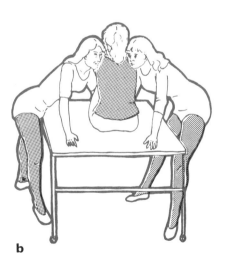

b

Fig. 3 The shoulder or Australian lift, showing position of patient (a) and of lifters (b).

of a lunge carry him/her **backwards** up the bed. The lifting movement should be rhythmical, smooth and continuous.

NOTE. The two lifters **must** press in towards each other. If the patient is **carried** any distance the lifters' free hands support the patient's back, e.g. when moving the patient from bed to chair.

2

2.3
Traditional, orthodox or cradle lift (2 lifters)

Common uses
Moving a patient up or down the bed.
Moving a patient from bed to chair.

Traditional lift up the bed
Position of the patient. Sitting with legs extended or flexed with arms crossed over his chest or round the lifters' neck and shoulders.

Position of the lifters. Wide base standing, facing each other at the sides of the bed and close in to the patient (see Fig. 4). The lifters' leading feet should point in the direction of movement. The lifters' hips and knees are flexed to the optimum position for a firm and secure grasp.

Grasp. Under the patient's upper thighs and over

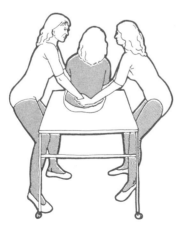

Fig. 4 Traditional, orthodox or cradle lift to move a patient up or down a bed or trolley.

the sacrum, with the lifters' elbows flexed and close into their sides. Wrist grasps can be used if suitable otherwise adapt.

The lift. To the command **'Ready—Lift'** the patient is lifted **up** off the bed. The lifters' hips and knees are extended and the patient is moved **upwards or downwards** by means of a lunge on to the leading foot. The whole lifting procedure should be rhythmical, smooth and continuous.

NOTE. Lifting a patient from bed or trolley to chair is shown in Fig. 5 (a, side view; b, front view; and c, in transit).

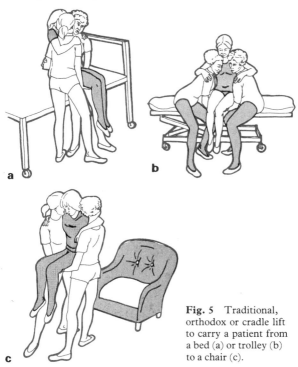

Fig. 5 Traditional, orthodox or cradle lift to carry a patient from a bed (a) or trolley (b) to a chair (c).

2.4
Stretcher or trolley lift (3 lifters)

Lifting a patient from bed to trolley

Position of the patient. Lying flat in bed with the head supported by one pillow and the arms across the abdomen.

Position of the trolley. In alignment with the foot of the bed. The brakes of the bed and the trolley must be in the locked position.

Position of the lifters. They are all on the same side of the bed standing with a fairly wide base with the leading foot of each pointing in the direction of movement.

Grasps. Lifter No. 1   Arms underneath the patient's head and shoulders.

Lifter No. 2   Arms underneath the patient's thighs and pelvis.

NOTE. This operator is the leading lifter and gives the command or signal to lift.

Lifter No. 3   Arms under the patient's legs.

The lift. To the chosen command the patient is gently pulled forwards on the bed. The operators then **lift** (keeping their elbows flexed, and close to their sides) by extending their hips and knees. Where possible, the patient is then rolled towards the lifters' chests and carried in this position (usually feet first). On reaching the trolley, the lifters' position and stabilise their stance before lowering the patient.

3
Technical Nursing Procedures

3

3.1
Taking and recording of temperature, pulse and respiration (TPR)

3

Temperature is the degree of warmth or coldness of a substance, compared with a recognised standard. A patient's body temperature is recorded by means of a clinical thermometer and the Celsius/Centigrade scale is used (for taking and recording temperature of children, see also Procedure 8.3).

Equipment
A tray containing:
Clinical thermometer
Steritemp sleeve or 2 Mediswabs to wipe thermometer before and after use
Watch with a second hand
Temperature chart
Pen
Box of tissues
Disposal bag

Procedures
There are four suitable sites to take a temperature, but as each gives a different result the same site must be used each time, for the same patient.
The sites are: in the mouth, axilla, groin and rectum.

1 *Taking a temperature in the mouth*
(a) Ascertain if this method is used in the area.
(b) Check the thermometer reading and shake down the mercury in the thermometer, if required. Apply the sleeve, if used, and place the bulb of the

thermometer under the centre of the patient's tongue.

(c) Instruct the patient to close his/her lips and not to bite the thermometer.

(d) Leave the thermometer in position for the recommended time.

(e) Remove the thermometer, wipe it, read it and record the temperature neatly on the chart. Check the temperature and shake down the mercury in the thermometer. Discard the sleeve if used.

Do **not** take an oral temperature:

If the patient is a child.

In delirious, unconscious, elderly or confused patients.

In epileptic, psychiatric, mentally handicapped patients or those who recently have had a myocardial infarction.

Where the patient has difficulty in breathing, particularly through his nose.

Immediately after the patient has had a hot or cold drink or after smoking.

2 *Taking a temperature in the axilla or groin.*

(a) Prepare the thermometer as in item 1(b) and ensure that the skin surfaces of the temperature site are dry.

(b) Place the thermometer in position with the bulb completely surrounded by skin and with no clothing intervening.

(c) Draw the patient's arm across his/her chest or cross one thigh over the other to hold the thermometer in position.

(d) Leave the thermometer in position for the recommended time.

(e) Remove and proceed as in item 1(e).

Do **not** take a temperature in the axilla or groin:

If the patient is very thin.

Immediately after the patient has had a bath or shower.

3 *Taking a temperature in the rectum.* A special thermometer is used with a shorter, rounded bulb and a jar of petroleum jelly is added to the tray.

The rectal method should be used for all infants and for adults where other methods are not possible. Rectal thermometers should be kept separate from other thermometers.

(a) Prepare the thermometer as 1(b) greasing the bulb with the lubricant, once the thermometer is in its sleeve.

(b) Gently insert the thermometer into the patient's rectum for 2–5 cm and hold it in position for the recommended time.

(c) Remove the thermometer and remove and discard the sleeve and proceed as in item 1(e).

The **pulse** is the wave of expansion and recoil occurring in an artery in response to the pumping action of the heart. The pulse is usually recorded by taking the radial pulse (for taking and recording pulse of children, see also Procedure 8.4).

Procedure

1 The patient must be lying in a relaxed position or sitting comfortably in a chair. His/her arm must be relaxed and supported.

2 Place the tips of the first three fingers along the line of the radial artery at the base of the patient's thumb with the index finger nearest to the palm of the patient's hand and the thumb at the back of the patients wrist. **Never** try to feel the pulse with your thumb as its own pulse may interfere with the reading.

3 When the patient's pulse is clearly felt count the number of beats in 1 minute using a watch with a second hand and immediately write down the result and note the volume and rhythm.

Respiration consists of an inspiration, expiration and pause and is normally rhythmical and quiet. It may be counted as the number of times the chest or upper abdomen rises in 1 minute (for counting and recording respiration in children, see also Procedure 8.4).

Procedure

1   The patient must be comfortably at rest before beginning to count respiration rate and the pulse.

2   **Do not** let the patient be aware of what you are doing, as it is possible to alter voluntarily the respiration rate. Do this by counting the rate whilst the fingers are on the patient's pulse.

3   Count the respirations for a full minute and immediately write down the result.

4   Whilst counting the respiration rate note the rhythm and depth of respiration. The normal rhythm is inspiration, expiration, pause. Any difficulty in breathing (dyspnoea) should be reported to the nurse in charge at once and the condition is usually relieved by supporting the patient in an upright position (see Procedure 1.6).

3.2
Taking an apex beat

3

Two nurses are essential for this procedure as both radial pulse and the apex beat **must be taken over the same minute.**

Equipment
Stethoscope
Watch with second hand
TPR chart

Procedure
1   The procedure is explained to the patient who should be in a relaxed position either sitting comfortably in a chair or upright in bed. Privacy is ensured.
2   The left half of the patient's chest is exposed and one nurse identifies the apex beat (it can normally be felt in the fifth intercostal space approximately in the mid-clavicular line) while the other identifies the radial pulse.
3   The watch is positioned so that both nurses can read it readily. The nurse recording the apex beat places the stethoscope over the appropriate spot and ensures she can hear the apex beat clearly. At a pre-arranged time the apex beat and the radial pulse are counted **over the same minute.**
4   The results are then neatly charted using different colours to denote each result and any deficit calculated.
5   The patient is made comfortable and the results are reported to the nurse in charge.

3.3
Taking and recording the arterial blood pressure

The blood pressure is the force of blood extended on the walls of the blood vessels through which it is flowing. It is the arterial blood pressure which is normally recorded.

Equipment
A sphygmomanometer (the cuff is selected appropriate to the arm size of the patient)
Stethoscope

Procedure
1   The patient should be mentally and physically at rest, seated or in bed.
2   The sphygmomanometer is placed on the bed or locker top at the same level as the patient's arm. Care should be taken to avoid the patient being able to read the mercury column whilst this procedure is being carried out.
3   The patient's arm is exposed and the cuff is wrapped evenly and firmly just above the patient's elbow (cubital fossa) and the tubing connected.
4   The valve is closed and the radial artery palpated. Air is then pumped into the cuff to a reading level on the mercury column of 20 mm above the level at which the radial pulse disappears.
5   The bell or diaphragm of the stethoscope is placed over the brachial artery and the valve gently released allowing the level of mercury to fall until the **first clear sound** is heard — this is the **systolic reading.**

6   The release of the valve continues until the **loud beats** give place to **muffled sounds**. The **point** at which this change occurs being taken as the **diastolic reading**. The sounds normally continue for a little longer before finally fading out altogether.

7   The tubing is disconnected and the cuff removed and the patient is made comfortable.

8   The readings are neatly charted.

NOTE. **Pulse pressure** is the difference between the systolic and diastolic pressure.

3.4
Starch poultice

3

A starch poultice has a cooling action in animal ringworm lesions and is useful for removing thick crusts in impetigo or other crusted lesions.

Equipment
Starch powder
Bowl
Cold water
Boiling water
Spoon
Linen—cut and cornered to size required
Gauze (to cover)
Spatula
Foil tray
Bandage—crimp or gauze
Disposal bag

Preparation
1½ tablespoons of starch powder to 285 ml of cold water is mixed to a thick, smooth cream in the bowl.
Boiling water is added continuously, stirring all the time until the starch changes colour from white to bluish white and thickens.
The consistency should be jelly like but not too stiff.
When cool spread 2 cm thick on the prepared linen.
The starch poultice may be covered with a thin layer of gauze.

Application
Apply and keep in place by a light crimp or gauze
bandage.

Removal
Removal in 4 to 6 hours.

3.5
Kaolin poultice (traditional)

3

A kaolin poultice is used to relieve pain and improve circulation.

Equipment
Tin of kaolin
Pot of boiling water
Spatula (in jug of hot water)
Wool pad
Linen—cut and cornered to size required
Gauze (to cover)
Foil tray
Bandage or binder
Disposal bag

Preparation
Kaolin is heated by **loosening the lid** and standing the tin in a pot of boiling water which is heated on a cooker. The kaolin is heated through by stirring intermittently with a spatula. The tin of kaolin is removed when heated and it is spread 0.5 cm thick evenly on the prepared linen. If being applied to the front of the chest a thickness of 0.25 cm is usually sufficient. The kaolin poultice may be covered with a thin layer of gauze.

Application
The kaolin poultice is taken to the patient's bedside in the foil tray and **tested for temperature before it is applied.** It is then placed gently on the

affected site, ensuring that the patient does not con-
sider it too hot, covered with a wool pad to retain
the heat and bandaged in position.

Renewed as prescribed

3

Kaolin poultice (K/L pack)

Equipment
K/L pack of kaolin poultice
Pot of boiling water
Gauze swabs (10 cm × 10 cm)
Bandage or binder
Scissors
Forceps
Foil tray
Disposal bag

Preparation
Drop one or more K/L packs as required into boiling water and leave for **not** more than 40 seconds.

Remove from heat using forceps and lay down pack with its metal foil side downwards.

Cut around the four edges of the pack and peel off the clear polythene layer.

Open out gauze swab/s and place over the kaolin pack **ensuring** that there is an overlap of 2.5 cm of gauze around all edges of the pack.

Application
As per Procedure 3.4 with the exception of covering the kaolin poultice with a wool pad. The foil backing of the pack helps to retain the heat in this instance.

Renewal
As per Procedure 3.4.

NOTE. 'Old' kaolin debris is removed from the

site of application by gently swabbing the affected area with olive oil and then by washing the area with warm soapy water. The affected area is then gently and carefully patted dry.

3

3.6
Administration of enemas

3

An enema is the introduction of a solution into the lower bowel. It may be used to evacuate the bowel or introduce drugs, e.g. steroids. Evacuant enemas include a disposable enema unit, enema saponis, arachis or olive oil.

3.7
Administration of a disposable evacuant enema unit

A disposable evacuant enema unit is pre-prepared and consists of a polythene bag with a nozzle attached and contains a specific action solution. Instructions for use **must** be read before use.

Equipment
As for Procedure 1.19 plus:
Enema unit standing in a jug of warm water (37.8°C)
Lotion thermometer
Lubricant
Medical wipes
Disposable bag
Waterproof protection for the bed
Disposal glove
    NOTE. If a commode is used the above equipment is used with the exception of a covered bedpan and a covered urinal for the male patient.

Preparation of the patient
Explain each step of the procedure to the patient to gain his cooperation.

Procedure
1   Ensure complete privacy for the patient and help him/her to relax.
2   Turn back the top bed clothes and place the patient in the left lateral position and cover his/her shoulders and back warmly.
3   Suitably arrange the patient's bed-wear and pro-

tect the bed by placing the waterproof sheeting under the patient's buttocks.

4   Remove enema unit from warm water and check instructions for administration. Put on the disposable glove. Remove seal from end of nozzle of enema unit and squeeze pack to expel air. Lubricate the nozzle before gently inserting it into the patient's rectum for 7–10 cm. Give the enema slowly over a period of 5 minutes so allowing the faeces to soften.

5   Slowly withdraw the nozzle and discard the unit and glove.

6   Encourage the patient to rest and retain the fluid for at least 5 minutes if possible.

7   If bedpan is used, proceed as per Procedure 1.19, items 3–11 inclusive.

If a commode is used, proceed as per Procedure 1.21, items 3–11 inclusive.

Aftercare of equipment
If a bedpan is used, as per Procedure 1.19.
If a commode is used, as per Procedure 1.21.
  NOTE. Wash hands **thoroughly**.

Observation and reporting
As per Procedure 1.18.

3.8
Administration of evacuant enema (enema saponis)

Equipment
As for Procedure 3.7 plus:
A large bowl containing tubing, funnel and connections already assembled
Disposable rectal catheter of a size suitable to the patient
Jug of solution (100 ml of soap solution in 400 ml of water at 37.8°C
which is mixed carefully to avoid air bubbles in the solution)
Disposable glove

Preparation of the patient
As per Procedure 3.7.

Procedure
1 As per Procedure 3.7 items 1–3 inclusive
2 Test the temperature of the solution. Put on disposable glove.
3 Using the assembled apparatus lubricate the catheter and run through a small amount of the solution to expel air. Nip the catheter and gently insert into the patient's rectum for 7–10 cm.
4 Run the fluid in evenly and at a low pressure preventing the entry of air by keeping the funnel full.
5 When the desired amount has been given pinch the tube and remove the catheter gently and

slowly, putting the apparatus back in the large bowl. Discard the glove.

6   Encourage the patient to retain the fluid for 5–10 minutes.

7   If a bedpan is used, proceed as per Procedure 1.19, items 3–11 inclusive.

If a commode is used, proceed as per Procedure 1.21, items 3–11 inclusive.

Aftercare of equipment
If a bedpan is used, as per Procedure 1.19.
If a commode is used, as per Procedure 1.21.
Plus thorough washing and cleaning of all non-disposable equipment used with detergent and hot water and/or recommended disinfectant.
NOTE. Wash hands **thoroughly**.

Observation and reporting
As per Procedure 1.18.

Paediatric nursing notes
The **correct size of catheter** to use in the administration of enema in children depends on the child's age and size. Always check the size of catheter with the nurse in charge of the ward.

The **amount of enema solution** for a child is approximately 30 ml per year of life until adult amount of 500 ml is reached. Always check with the nurse in charge of the ward the correct amount of fluid to be administered.

3.9
Olive or arachis oil enema

Equipment as for disposable enema unit (see Procedure 3.7) and prepared as for evacuant type.

120–180 ml (see Procedure 3.8) of warm olive or arachis oil (37.8°C) is given slowly should be retained for 4 hours.

The foot of the bed is elevated if the patient's condition allows to assist in the retention of the fluid.

The olive or arachis oil enema on expiry of the retention time is followed by an evacuant enema.

3.10
Steroid retention enema

3

A steroid retention enema is given for ulcerative colitis. It is a disposable pack retention enema which should be prepared, checked and administered as directed by the instructions on the pack which are similar to those for the disposable evacuant enema unit, but in this instance the solution is retained.

3.11
Administration of an evacuant suppository

3

A rectal evacuant suppository is a small cone or torpedo-shaped object with medicant added to a base which may be made of gelatine, wax or cocoa butter. It dissolves at bowel heat and becomes active, producing an evacuation in normally 20–60 minutes.

Equipment
Suppository as per prescription sheet
Lubricant or gallipot with warm water (37.8°C)
Disposable towel
Medical wipes
Disposable glove or finger cot
Disposal bag

Preparation of the patient
As for an evacuant enema (see Procedure 3.8) except that it is essential to explain to the patient that it may take from half to several hours to stimulate defaecation. Reassure the patient that a bedpan or commode will be given when requested.

Procedure
1 Identify the patient with the name on the prescription and medicine recording sheets and the patient's identiband.
2 Proceed as per Procedure 3.7 items 1–3 inclusive with the exception that in this instance the bed is protected by the disposable towel.

3   Remove outer cover from the suppository and dip the suppository into the warm water or apply lubricant as indicated (after carefully reading the instruction for administration).

4   Put on disposable glove or finger cot and using the index finger gently insert the suppository, pointed end first, into the patient's rectum until the anal sphincter grips the second phalangeal joint.

5   Withdraw index finger carefully and discard glove or cot.

6   Encourage the patient to retain the suppository for as long as possible.

7   Leave the patient comfortable with instruction how to call for assistance when required.

8   Remove screens and clear away equipment.

Aftercare of equipment

Place disposable bag and contents into appropriate container.

Wash and dry all non-disposable equipment.

Wash hands thoroughly and record administration of the suppository on the medicine recording sheet.

Aftercare of patient and subsequent equipment

If a bedpan is used as per Procedure 1.19.

If a commode is used as per Procedure 1.21.

Observation and reporting

As per Procedure 1.18.

3.12
Rectal lavage (adult)

Rectal lavage is the washing out of the rectum to prepare the patient's lower bowel prior to certain examinations or operations (for rectal and colonic lavage in children, see Procedure 8.6 and 8.7). An evacuant enema may be given 30–60 minutes before a rectal lavage.

Equipment
Trolley with:
Waterproof protection for the bed and the floor
Disposable rectal catheter of a size suitable to the
    patient
Funnel, tubing and connection/s already assembled
Lubricant
Medical wipes
Lotion thermometer
Large jugs with warm water (37.8°C)
Bucket for returned fluid
Disposal glove
Disposable bag

Preparation of patient
Explain each step of the procedure to the patient and gain his/her cooperation. Give reassurance as required.

Procedure
1   As per Procedure 3.7, items 1–3 inclusive.
2   Place waterproof covering and bucket on the floor at the side of the bed.

3 Test the temperature of the water. Put on the disposable glove.

4 Using the assembled apparatus lubricate the catheter and run through a small amount of water to expel the air. Nip the catheter and gently insert into the patient's rectum for 7–10 cm.

5 Run the fluid in evenly into the rectum **giving no more than 300 ml at a time**. Before the funnel is empty invert the funnel over the bucket and allow the fluid to drain back.

6 Repeat the process in item 5 until the return fluid is clear.

7 Gently remove the catheter and measure the amount of fluid given and returned

8 Remove equipment and leave the patient comfortable.

NOTE. The patient may require a bedpan or commode at the end of this procedure.

Aftercare of equipment
Place disposal bag and contents into appropriate container.
Thoroughly wash and clean all non-disposable equipment.
Wash hands thoroughly.

Observation and reporting
Note and report any discomfort or pain the patient may have during the procedure.
Inspect contents of the bucket before disposal and report same.

3.13
Preoperative care—general notes

3

Preparation of the patient

1 Ensure the patient understands the nature of the operation.

2 Liaise with relatives regarding visiting, etc.

3 Explain preoperative and postoperative care to the patient, reassure frequently.

5 Preoperative skin shave (if required) and bath.

6 Suppository or enema preoperative evening (as prescribed).

7 Fast patient from designated time as appropriate.

8 **Morning of operation**

(a) **Check patient's identity** verbally and against case notes, i.e. patient's full name and age.

(b) Remove all patient's jewellery into safe keeping (wedding ring may be taped to patient's finger), denture(s) and prostheses are also removed being placed in an appropriate named container. If patient uses a hearing aid, it is labelled, and if required, accompanies patient to theatre.

(c) Patient should empty bladder unless otherwise instructed.

(d) Assist the patient to put on cap, gown and socks, ensuring the bed is appropriately prepared.

(e) Ensure any instructions from medical staff are carried out, e.g. premedication, catheterisation, nasogastric intubation.

(f) Ensure all appropriate documents are in order, and are sent to theatre with patient, e.g.
consent form, duly signed
case notes

x-rays

medicine prescription and recording sheets with temperature, pulse, respiration and blood pressure clearly marked

(g) Nurse and porter transfer the patient to the Theatre Suite.

(h) **Further patient identity check** with theatre nurse.

(i) Prepare patient's bed and equipment required in readiness for his return from theatre.

(j) Prepare appropriate recording charts for patient's return from theatre.

3.14
Preoperative check list

3

1   Patient's name in full and age

2   Registration number (on identity wristband clearly)

3   Consent form for operation and anaesthesia duly signed.

4   Remove all jewellery (wedding ring may be taped), denture(s) and prostheses. Hearing aid, if needed, should accompany patient and its safety ensured.

5   All makeup and hair clips removed.

6   Gown, cap and socks.

7   Allergies, e.g. elastoplast, drugs, etc. noted.

8   Routine urinalysis obtained and recorded.

9   Weight recorded.

10   Time of last meal or drink.

11   Recording sheets with current temperature, pulse, respiration and blood pressure clearly marked.

12   Medicine prescription with premedication time entered as appropriate.

13   X-rays.

14   Case notes.

15   Ensure patient's safety during transportation to theatre suite.

16   **Check details** on arrival at theatre, with theatre nurse.

3.15
Postoperative care—general notes

3

1   Patient is transferred into a warm bed from the trolley.

2   If patient is still unconscious, **maintain a clear airway**.

3   Place the patient in an appropriate position according to the operation and the anaesthetists instructions.

4   Commence administration of oxygen, as per instruction.

5   **Check** any intravenous infusion/transfusion.

6   **Check** wounds and drains.

7   Whilst the patient is unconscious 15-minute interval recordings of pulse, respiration rate and blood pressure are made.

8   Leave capable nurse in charge of the patient and instruct her/him to report immediately any abnormal recordings or change in the patient's condition. Give an accurate verbal report to the nurse in charge of the ward, e.g.

   operation performed
   condition of the patient
   pulse, respiration and blood pressure
   drains, packs, urinary catheter in situ
   intravenous fluid therapy
   sedation/analgesic, if any, administered
   if patient's throat sprayed with anaesthetic

9   Observe the patient closely until conscious.

10   Ensure the withholding of oral fluids, where necessary, e.g. after local anaesthetic to the throat or major surgery.

11   Ensure accurate measurement and observation of fluid intake and output—report any abnormalities.

12   Record pulse, blood pressure, respiration rate and temperature as instructed—report any abnormalities.

13   Ensure patient's maximum comfort and carry out general nursing care.

14   Encourage the patient to carry out breathing and limb exercises.

15   Ensure early ambulation whenever possible.

POSTOPERATIVE NURSING CARE FOR SPINAL OR EPIDURAL ANAESTHESIA

1   Care of the lower limbs in the absence of sensation.

2   Careful recording of the patient's blood pressure and pulse—danger of hypotension.

3   All patients have intravenous infusion in progress.

4   Report any patient's headache or delay of sensation returning to the lower limbs to the nurse in charge.

3.16
Preparation and use of a basic trolley for sterile procedures

Preparation and equipment

1   Carefully wash and dry hands.

2   Swab both shelves (upper shelf first) and bars of the trolley with the recommended lotion.

3   Place the following items in an orderly manner on the lower shelf:

small dressing pack (containing gauze swabs, gallipot, wool balls, drape and 3 sets of forceps)

scissor set

skin cleansing lotion

material to secure dressing/s, e.g. zinc oxide strapping, bandages, elastoplast, micropore

4   Mask/s.

5   Disposal bag.

6   **Plus** additional items as required for specific procedures, e.g. sterile gloves.

Procedure

During the procedure the **dresser** is the nurse carrying out the procedure and the **assistant** is the nurse helping with the procedure.

1   **Assistant** (masked) washes hands and dries them on a **clean** paper towel, then opens the dressing pack by tearing across the top of its outer envelope. Then either shakes the inner pack on to the centre of the upper shelf of the trolley **or** allows the **dresser** (masked and having washed hands) to remove it.

2   The **dresser** carefully opens out the inner pack

so as to allow its **inner surface** to be used as a **sterile area.**

3   The **assistant** opens and carefully tips the contents of any other sterile packs requested by the **dresser** on to the **sterile working area. (No unsterile parts must touch this area.)**

4   The **assistant** pours lotions into sterile gallipots as instructed by the **dresser**.

5   Throughout the procedure both the **assistant** and the **dresser** are responsible for the general welfare of the patient. Most supportive care is usually given by the **assistant**.

Aftercare of equipment

Disposal bag and its contents (soiled dressing swabs, etc.) are placed in the appropriate container.

Unused packs and other materials from lower shelf are returned to their appropriate storage units.

The trolley is thoroughly cleaned with hot water and detergent and/or recommended disinfectant.

NOTE. Certain instruments are returned to the Central Sterile Supply Department (CSSD) after use.

This basic trolley can be used for all minor surgical procedures, including dressings at ward and departmental level.

3.17
Wound dressing

A wound is a break in the continuity of parts of the body—skin, mucous membranes, muscle tendons, etc.—and may either be superficial or deep. It can be accidental or intentional.

Approximately 50% of patient's have some form of wound.

Complete asepsis must be observed in caring for all types of wounds by employing a **non-touch aseptic technique,** by the use of sterile instruments and dressings.

Order of doing dressings
1   Clean wounds.
2   Potentially infected wounds, e.g. wounds in known contaminated areas: where there is any type of drainage; burns; ulcers.
3   Infected wounds.

Wound dressings should be carried out in a treatment room and no other activities should take place in the room while the dressings are in progress.

When dressings are done in the open ward, these should **not be** done immediately after bedmaking or ward cleaning.

Non-touch aseptic technique **must** always be used. The trolley **must** be freshly prepared between each dressing.

Where possible dressings are always done by two nurses. A **dresser** and an **assistant** (see Procedure 3.16 for definition).

3

Preparation of the patient

1   Explain the procedure to the patient and afford reassurance.

2   Ensure privacy.

3   Position the patient and arrange bed clothes according to the wound area, e.g. abdominal wounds, if possible, remove all but one pillow and ask the patient to place his/her arms by his/her sides.

4   Ensure warmth and general comfort for the patient.

Procedure

1   Both the **assistant** and the **dresser**:
    put on mask
    wash and dry hands
    prepare the trolley

2   **Assistant:**

(a) Takes the trolley to patient's bedside.

(b) Removes outer dressing. Adhesive preparations are loosened by gentle pressure on the skin beneath the adhesive with one hand slowly pulling off the preparation with the other hand. A swab with appropriate plaster remover placed on the adhesive strands will assist in their removal.

(c) Washes hands again and dries them on a *clean* paper towel. A swab or specimen of exudate may be taken by assistant if required.

(d) Opens packets as requested.

(e) Pours out lotion/s.

(f) Generally assists the **dresser** and helps to reassure the patient.

3   **Dresser:**

(a) Washes hands and forearms thoroughly and dries them on a *clean* paper towel.

(b) Using non-touch aseptic technique arranges sterile equipment in order of use on upper shelf of

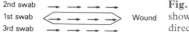

Fig. 6 Wound showing order and direction of swabs.

the trolley, creating a sterile working area.

(c) Removes soiled dressing with forceps and places in disposal bag or soiled dressing container.

(d) With other two pairs of forceps:

    (i) drapes wound area with sterile drape/s

    (ii) swabs wound as illustrated in figure 6 with slightly moistened swabs, using a swab **once only**. This is repeated with dry swabs.

    NOTE. Additional swabbing may be required if there is excessive discharge or crusting. Clean, incised wounds should have the **minimum** of swabbing.

    (iii) Proceed with dressing, as per instructions.

    (iv) Cover wound adequately with final dressing and secure with appropriate material. Before securing a dressing it may be necessary to remove traces of adhesive materials from the previous dressing with appropriate plaster remover.

(e) Report condition of patient's wound and general condition.

4   Both the **assistant** and the **dresser**:

    re-arrange bed clothes and pillows and leave the patient comfortable

    remove screens and remove and clear the trolley

After care of equipment

As per Procedure 3.16.

Special nursing note

When dealing with infected wounds, the **dresser** removes the soiled dressing as per item 3(c) of this procedure.

With other forceps the wound is covered with a swab (or swabs) while the surrounding areas are cleaned.

The trolley is cleaned and reset and the wound dressed as per item 3(d). All unused equipment, e.g. swabs, are discarded in this instance because of the possibility of cross-infection. Non-disposable equipment is thoroughly washed and cleaned with detergent and hot water and/or recommended disinfectant.

Infected wounds may be required to be dressed every 4 hours.

3.18
Specific notes for wound dressing

Removal of interrupted sutures

Interrupted sutures are a series of separate sutures
(see Fig. 7) and their removal is detailed in Figure
8.

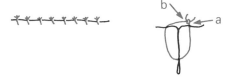

Fig. 7   (*left*) Interrupted sutures.

Fig. 8   (*right*) Removal of interrupted sutures: (a) point at which
suture is gently pulled away from the skin and cut as close to the
skin as possible; and (b) point at which suture is grasped with
the forceps and gently pulled out of the skin.

An end of a suture at *a* is grasped with the forceps
and gently pulled away from the skin. The tip of the
scissors (or stitch cutter) is passed under the drawn
up portion as **close** to the skin as possible and the
suture snipped (cut) At *b* gently pull out the suture
with the forceps.

NOTE. The portion of the suture on the surface
(i.e. external) **must not** be drawn through the
wound.

Alternative sutures should be removed first.
When this is done, it can be noted if there is good
union between the skin edges. If the union is good
the remainder of the sutures may be removed unless
otherwise instructed.

3

Removal of continuous sutures

Continuous sutures are formed from one length of thread and are of various types each requiring different techniques of removal.

One type is completely pulled through the wound after cutting it from its anchorage at either end of the wound.

Another type is removed by cutting the skin edge of each loop and removing as for an interrupted suture.

One form of subcuticular suture dissolves spontaneously with time and only the exposed portions are removed if necessary.

Another non-disposable type requires a knot to be removed from one end and is withdrawn by pulling from the other end.

Removal of Michel's clips

A Michel clip is removed by passing the curved, lower blade of the clip remover under the centre of the clip then bringing the two blades together. This frees the clip edges and the clip is then gently lifted off with forceps (see Fig. 9).

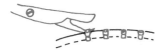

Fig. 9 Removal of Michel's clips, showing the position of the upper blade of the clip remover in the clip.

Removal of Avlox clips

The remover has a rocker action which opens the blades when pressure is applied on the handles thus releasing the clip (see Fig. 10).

Probing a wound

Probing a wound may be necessary when the

Fig. 10   Removal of Avlox clips, showing (*left*) the introduction of the clip remover and (*right*) the subsequent removal of the clip.

superficial layers are healing too quickly and, in consequence, allowing pocketing of exudate to occur. To prevent this a probe or sinus forceps may be inserted into the wound to open a tract to allow drainage to continue.

Suction drainage
Suction drainage is a form of closed drainage used to drain areas where a cavity has been left, e.g. after a mastectomy.

Application of Jelonet
After wound swabbing, a piece of jelonet of appropriate size to the wound is removed from its container using non-touch technique and applied to the wound area **only** so that it is completely covered. Other preparations of this type require medical prescription.

Application of powders
Powders may be dusted or insufflated on to the wound as per medical prescription.

Application of sprays from aerosols
Sprays are applied per medical prescription. Hold the aerosol approximately 30 cm from the wound and liberally spray. If being applied to the head or face cover the patient's eyes and ears.

Wound drains
Examples of types of drains are:
Circular rubber or plastic
Corrugated rubber
Paul's tubing (fine rubber)
Catheter, e.g. intrapleural
Closed—suction of an open wound

Shortening of a drain. Clean the wound and re-move remaining suture if present.
1 Gently rotate the drain to break any adhesions.
2 Withdraw 2.5 cm (or as instructed).
3 Insert fresh sterile safety pin a little below the point where the drain is to be put.
4 Clean round the drain then cut off the portion of the drain that is to be removed.
5 Swab the area and surround with gauze dressings and secure.

Removal of a drain. A drain may be situated in the main wound or through a separate stab incision. If a stab incision, the main wound is not disturbed.
1 Gently loosen pack from wound edges.
2 Cut and remove the drain's retaining suture.
3 Remove the drain slowly with forceps.
4 Ensure that all packs are removed.

Nursing note
If a 'T' tube is being removed it **must** be done by withdrawing it carefully as it is possible that it may break at the 'T' junction. If any difficulty (resistance) is experienced during withdrawal **stop** immediately and inform the medical staff.
An alternative catheter type of drain may be in situ, this makes withdrawal simpler.
    NOTE. For a wound dressing using the Hampshire dressing see Procedure 8.8.

3.19
Principles of bandaging

1 Use a tightly rolled bandage of suitable width and material.

2 Support the part being bandaged.

3 Face the patient when bandaging an arm or a leg.

4 Hold the head of the bandage uppermost.

5 Hold the bandage in the right hand when bandaging a left limb and vice versa.

6 Bandage a limb from within outwards and from below upwards, maintaining an even pressure throughout.

7 Begin the bandage with a secure turn and allow each turn to cover two-thirds of the preceding one.

8 **Ensure** that the bandage is neither too tight nor too loose.

9 Finish off the bandage with a straight turn fold in the end and secure, avoiding joints and the site of injury.

10 Fastening is normally with safety pins or the fastener provided with some bandages. **Zinc oxide tape is always used** in the confused, psychiatric, mentally handicapped or paediatric patient.

3.20
Principles of barrier nursing

Barrier nursing is a technique which entails the patient being nursed in an environment of isolation because of a potential infection or communicable disease and is thus prevented from infecting others. The isolation facilities required are determined by the degree of isolation found to be necessary.

It is used to minimise cross-infection by respiratory/droplet spread or faecal/oral spread.

Equipment
Protective clothing including:
Gowns
Masks
   rarely as routine
   reverse barrier nursing
   high risk nursing as a protection to wearer (filter type)
Gloves
   handling infected sites or materials
Footwear
   high risk nursing

Principles
Handwashing
Disinfection and safe disposal of articles
Terminal cleaning and disinfection of the patient's area.

Open ward barrier nursing
In open ward barrier nursing the principles are

applied to every patient. The success is dependent on the efficiency with which the technique is carried out by **all** staff. Wearing of barrier gowns and hand-washing before and after every service to the patient must be strictly adhered to.

General ward isolation
In a general ward isolation one or two patients are preferably barrier nursed in a side room with hand-washing facilities or in a corner of the ward adjacent to a washhand basin and service areas to which sanitary utensils can be taken by the shortest route. This would only be a **temporary measure** before transferring the patients to an isolation unit.

Cubicle isolation
In complete isolation the bedrooms are contained within an inner closed clean corridor and an open outer corridor for used articles. Filtered, heated air is pumped into the clean corridor, passes into the rooms and is withdrawn by an extractor fan placed in the roof of each bathroom annexe. All services move from the clean to the open outer corridor. All articles for the patient's use are kept in the room. Handwashing and gown facilities are provided in the vestibule of each bedroom for staff. **Isolation in a cubicle is not enough to eliminate cross-infection** but **must** be accompanied by good discipline and **strict barrier nursing technique**.

Barrier gown
It is most important while attending to or working in the vicinity of the patient that the barrier gown is **worn properly**. It must be understood that the outside of the gown is contaminated while the inside which comes into contact with the uniform is clean.

Gowns are kept on coat hangers right side out and should hang on a rail front to front.

Putting on the gown. The coat hanger hook is taken in the right hand and held with the back opening of the gown towards the nurse. The left arm is slipped into the gown and the coat hanger is transferred to the left hand and the right sleeve of the gown put on. The coat hanger is returned to the rail and the nurse fastens up the gown **properly** at the neck and waist.

Taking off the gown. Once the service to the patient has been completed the gown must be removed **without** contaminating the interior. The gown is unfastened at the neck and waist. The coat hanger is taken in the right hand, inserted at the neck into the left sleeve and the left arm is carefully withdrawn **without** touching the outside of the gown. The coat hanger is transferred to the left hand, the free end inserted into the right sleeve and the right arm similarly withdrawn. The hanger is then put on the rail correctly. **The hands are now thoroughly washed and dried.**

3.21
Administration of oxygen

3

Precautions
Oxygen is administered according to doctor's written instructions and **may only be administered** on a nurse's own initiative in an emergency.

Oxygen supports combustion, therefore all articles likely to cause sparks or flare **must be** removed from the immediate area, i.e.:

naked flames, e.g. matches, cigarette lighters, cigarettes and pipes

electrical equipment, e.g. electric shaver

clockwork toys, e.g. friction driven cars (also battery operated toys)

nylon materials, e.g. pyjamas or nightdress and bed clothing

A notice **OXYGEN—NO SMOKING must** be displayed for the attention of, in the main, visitors and other patients.

Equipment
Oxygen is administered from either an oxygen cylinder (coloured black with white upper part marked *oxygen*) or piped oxygen tubing.
These may be used with:

an appropriate mask, e.g. Ventimask

nasal cannulae and nasal cleaning equipment

oxygen tent

Procedures 8.11 and 8.12

incubator

respirator/ventilator

NOTE. Oxygen can also be given via tracheostomy to patients who do not require Intermittent Positive Pressure Ventilation (IPPV), e.g. laryngectomy.

Procedure

1   The procedure must first be explained to the patient and that it will help him/her to breathe more easily. The precautions associated with the administration of oxygen are also explained to the patient.

2   The tubing is connected to the cylinder or pipeline and the appropriate mask is connected to the other end of the tubing.

3   **Piped oxygen** is turned on by means of a control knob and regulated with a flow meter. **Oxygen cylinders** are turned on by turning the key three full turns anticlockwise then by the control knob attached to the flow meter which regulates the flow of oxygen.

4   Oxygen mask is applied over the patient's nose and mouth and is held in place by an elastic band which fits round the patient's head.

NOTE. **The flow of oxygen** is usually 4 litres per minute but this will depend upon the doctor's prescription.

Some means of **humidification** of oxygen may be necessary. Humidification is **always** used in the administration of oxygen by nasal cannulae. Sterile water should always be used in humidifiers.

Nasal cannulae

1   The patient's nostrils are first cleaned with cotton wool buds and water.

2   The nasal cannulae consists of a continuous piece of tubing terminating in two small cannulae which are inserted one just inside each nostril.

3   The rate of flow in this instance is usually 2 litres

per minute but this will depend on the doctor's prescription.

NOTE. *Therapeutic nebulisers* are **only** used on doctor's prescription.

Oxygen tents and incubators. Oxygen tents and incubators are mostly used for children and babies as they obviously will not keep an oxygen mask on. The child's hooded type of oxygen tent is called a croupette. (See Procedures 8.11 and 8.12.)

1   The oxygen tent is hooked on to the top and bottom of the bed and tucked under the mattress.

2   Both incubators and oxygen tents have either refrigeration or compartments for ice and distilled water to keep the oxygen cool and humid.

3   Before use the fine adjustment for oxygen flow **must be** opened before the main flow tap is turned on. Oxygen tents and incubators are **flushed first** with oxygen before the rate of flow is regulated.

3.22
Midstream specimen of urine

3

Equipment
Sterile bowl
Bedpan/urinal/toilet
Labelled sterile universal container
Bacteriology form

Preparation of the patient
Explain each step of the procedure to the patient
and gain his/her cooperation.

Procedure
1   Ensure privacy and cleanliness.
2   Place the bedpan under the patient, or give
urinal, or allow to the toilet.
3   Ask the patient to pass a small amount of urine
into the toilet receptacle, to stop the flow and then to
continue to pass urine into the sterile bowl. Remove
the bowl when sufficient urine has been collected,
taking care not to touch the inside or the rim of the
sterile bowl. Allow the patient to finish micturating.
4   Remove toilet receptacle. Make sure the patient
is dry and comfortable. Allow the patient to wash
his/her hands.
5   The urine from the sterile bowl is carefully
poured into the labelled sterile universal container
and sent to the bacteriology department with the
completed form as soon as possible after collection—if not refrigerate but **do not** freeze in the
refrigerator supplied for this purpose.
   NOTE. For the **dip slide method** see Procedure
8.5.

3.23
Urinary catheterisation

It must be stressed that urinary catheterisation should **only** be carried out when absolutely necessary because of the danger of urinary tract infections which may eventually lead to kidney failure.

Cleanliness of the patient **must be** ascertained before commencing the procedure. It is often advisable to bath the patient prior to catheterisation.

Equipment
Basic trolley for sterile procedures (see Procedure 3.16) plus:
Urinary catheter(s) appropriate size and type
Sterile bowl
Packet of drapes
Lubricant (local anaesthetic is included in the lubricant for the male patient)
2 pairs of sterile gloves
For an indwelling urinary catheter the following are also required:
20 ml syringe (no needle required)
30 ml of sterile fluid (normal saline 0.9% is used for Foley's catheters)
Drainage bag and holder
Tube clip (gate clip) if required
A specimen container may be required.

NOTE. Catheterisation packs are available and generally contain: container for urine; waterproof underpad; gloves; drape with aperture; forceps; gallipot; cotton wool balls; cleansing lotion; swabs; specimen container and disposal bag.

3

Preparation of the patient

Explain the procedure to the patient and ensure privacy.

Fold down the bed clothes and place the patient comfortably in the recumbent position with knees flexed apart.

Ensure that the patient's chest is covered.

A waterproof pillow may be placed under the patient's buttocks, if desired.

Procedure

Should be carried out by two nurses if possible.

1 Mask.

2 Wash and dry hands.

3 Take prepared trolley to the patient's bedside.

4 Open dressing pack and create a sterile field (area)

5 Open catheter pack covering and any other packs required and **without** allowing unsterile parts to come into contact with the sterile area carefully drop the equipment on to this area.

6 Open lubricant and **very carefully** squeeze some of the lubricant on to one of the sterile swabs ready for lubricating the catheter.

7 Put on sterile gloves and arrange equipment on the sterile area.

8 Pour cleansing lotion.

9 Place drapes in position.

Female patient. (a) Part the labia majora with two dry swabs and using the index finger and thumb draw the labia majora upwards and expose and part the labia minora.

(b) Swab the labia clean working from outside inwards and from above downwards. Use each swab **once only** and discard.

(c) Dry the area with a cotton wool ball and remove

117

the two dry swabs.

(d) Remove and discard gloves. Put on the second pair of sterile gloves and lubricate the catheter and leave ready.

(e) Part the labia using a sterile swab and using forceps gently swab the external urethral opening (meatus).

(f) Place urine container (bowl) in position.

(g) Take the catheter in the **sterile hand** and gently introduce the catheter into the urethral orifice without touching the labia. Allowing the free end of the catheter to drop into the urine container (bowl). (If any resistance is met, stop the procedure immediately and report to the nurse in charge.)

Male patient. Urinary catheterisation in the male patient is done by a doctor or a male nurse.

(a) Gently push back the prepuce to expose the glans penis using a dry swab.

(b) Wrap a swab round the penis and swab the glans penis in a backward direction from the urethral meatus. Use each swab **once only** and discard.

(c) Dry the area with a cotton wool ball.

(d) Remove and discard gloves. Put on second pair of sterile gloves and lubricate the catheter and leave ready.

(e) Place urine container (bowl) in position.

(f) Lift the patient's penis slightly and take the catheter in the **sterile hand** and gently introduce the catheter into the urethral orifice, allowing the free end of the catheter to drop into the urine container (bowl). (If any resistance is met, stop immediately and report to the nurse in charge.)

(g) The prepuce must be pushed back over the glans penis after catheterisation.

10 Note the urinary flow and obtain specimen if required.

11 **Either:** withdraw the catheter once the bladder is decompressed **or** inflate the catheter balloon using the amount of sterile fluid specified. (See retention catheter.)

12 Clear away equipment and make the patient comfortable.

13 Unscreen the bed and remove the trolley.

Special nursing notes

If the catheter becomes unsterile during any part of the procedure discard and use another.

It is important, especially in cases of urinary retention that the urinary bladder is slowly decompressed.

Length of urethra:
  female 4–5 cm
  male 15–20 cm

Aftercare of equipment

As per Procedure 3.16.

Observations and reporting

Report on the amount of urine obtained and any abnormalities.

Check that the specimen is properly labelled and send it immediately with the appropriate form to the bacteriology department.

Retention catheter

A retention catheter has an inflatable bag (balloon) at its distal end and a side arm extension at its proximal end.

Sterile fluid is injected (without a needle) into the

3

valve in the side arm extension to inflate the balloon.

The open end of the retention catheter is attached to a drainage bag.

A tube clip may be used.

The size of the retention catheter and the amount of fluid introduced is noted in the nursing Kardex.

Complications of catheterisation
Introduction of infection

Damage to the urethra

Loss of bladder control

NOTE. Spigots are **only** used to close the inlet tube where bladder irrigation is discontinued.

3.24
Care of an indwelling (retention) urinary catheter

1 Make sure that the catheter is correctly positioned at all times and not kinked.

2 Swab the exposed part of the catheter once or twice daily with suitable disinfectant.

3 Rotate the catheter regularly to prevent adhesions forming.

4 In intermittent drainage a tube clip (gate clip) is used on the tubing.

5 Empty or change drainage bag regularly (night or morning or when full).

6 When bedmaking or turning or lifting the patient ensure that the drainage bag is **not** raised above the level of the patient's buttocks without the tubing being clipped off, so preventing backflow into the bladder.

7 Ensure an adequate fluid intake.

3.25
Catheter specimen of urine

3

A catheter specimen of urine may be required to obtain a urine specimen from a patient with an indwelling catheter in situ and a closed drainage system in operation.

Equipment
Tray with:
Sterile syringe and needle
Cleaning agent, e.g. Mediswabs
Tube clip (gate clip) or forceps
Labelled sterile universal container
Bacteriology form

Procedure
1   Explain the procedure to the patient and ensure privacy.
2   Clip the urine drainage bag tubing below the level of the self-sealing ring, having first ensured that any urine in the tubing has been drained into the bag.
3   Leave the tubing clipped off until there is sufficient fresh urine in the tube to obtain a specimen (10–30 minutes).
4   Wash and dry hands.
5   Using cleaning agent (Mediswab) clean the self-sealing strip on the tubing thoroughly.
6   A specimen may now be obtained with care using the needle and syringe.

7   Withdraw needle and release the clip to allow free drainage of urine to recommence.

8   Transfer the urine specimen to the sterile universal container and send it immediately with the appropriate form to the bacteriology department.

9   Make the patient comfortable, clear away equipment and unscreen the bed.

NOTE. For catheter specimen of urine in children see Procedure 8.5.

3.26
Removal of an indwelling (retention) urinary catheter

3

Equipment
Trolley or tray with:
A small dressing pack
A sachet of aqueous cleaning lotion
20 ml syringe
Bowl
Measuring jug
Protection for the bed (incontinence pad)
Disposal bag

Procedure
1   Ascertain from the nursing Kardex the amount of fluid in the retention catheter balloon.
2   Explain the procedure to the patient and ensure privacy and place an incontinence pad beneath the patient's buttocks.
3   Wash hands.
4   Drain the residual amount of urine from the catheter into the bowl and measure the amount.
5   Swab the area proximal to the external urethral opening (meatus) and dry gently.
6   Remove the fluid from the catheter balloon with the syringe by withdrawing the fluid through the valve connection in the side arm extension. Ensure that the amount withdrawn is equivalent to that stated in the nursing Kardex.
7   Remove the catheter by gentle traction. (Should any difficulty be experienced stop immediately and report to the nurse in charge.)

8   Clean and dry the area as before (item 5).

9   Leave the patient comfortable and explain how he/she can cooperate in regaining bladder control.

10   Clear away equipment and unscreen the bed.

11   Wash hands, complete the appropriate chart and report to the nurse in charge the result.

3

3.27
Bladder lavage

3

Bladder lavage is the washing out of urinary bladder with sterile fluid. It may be carried out:

> preoperatively to remove clots in bladder haemorrhage
>
> to cleanse the bladder with urinary disinfectants in some forms of urinary infections
>
> postoperatively for clot retention following prostatectomy

Equipment
Basic trolley for sterile procedure (see Procedure 3.16) plus:

50 ml bladder syringe with central nozzle

Lavage fluid, e.g. sterile aqueous chlorhexidine 1 in 5000 (0.02%) (labelled for bladder irrigation), standing in a jug of water at 37.8°C (other solutions may be ordered for washout)

Sterile gloves

2 sterile paper towels

2 sterile bowls (one to hold the lavage fluid and the other to collect urine and returned fluid)

Jug

Preparation of the patient
As per Procedure 3.17. The patient is likely to have a urinary catheter in situ.

Procedure
Where possible this procedure should be carried out by two nurses.

1 Wash and dry hands.
2 Mask.
3 Take the trolley to the patient's bedside.
4 Open sterile pack and prepare the trolley.
5 Place sterile towels in position.
6 Place bowl for return fluid on a paper towel.
Remove the urine bag from the catheter and discard.
Allow the catheter to drain into the bowl. Measure
and discard urine collected. Replace the bowl.
7 Fill the second sterile bowl with lavage solution.
Put on sterile gloves. Draw solution into the syringe
and inject the solution evenly and gently into the
urinary bladder through the catheter.
8 Remove the syringe and allow the fluid to drain
naturally from the bladder. Repeat until the washout is complete or the return fluid is clear.
9 If the fluid does not return naturally, aspirate
with the syringe. This may be necessary when blood
clots are present in the urinary bladder. (Sodium
citrate 0.5% may be prescribed by the doctor for
injection via the urinary catheter into the bladder to
assist in removal of blood clots.)
10 Affix new drainage bag to the catheter.
11 Clear away equipment, leave the patient comfortable and remove the screens.

Aftercare of equipment
As per Procedure 3.16 plus measuring the amount
of returned fluid.

Observations and reporting
Note the presence of any abnormalities in the returned fluid and report the result to the nurse in
charge.
Complete appropriate chart.

3.28
Continuous bladder irrigation

3

On rare occasions continuous bladder irrigation might be necessary to remove heavily contaminated material from a diseased urinary bladder.

It may also be necessary following a prostatectomy to remove blood clots.

Equipment
Basic trolley for sterile procedures (see Procedure 3.16) plus:
Disposable irrigation set
Sterile aqueous chlorhexidine 1 in 5000 (0.02%)
Infusion stand
Urine drainage bag with outlet valve on lower
  border

Procedure
The patient requires either a three-way urethral catheter or a suprapubic catheter and urethral catheter in situ.

1   Arrange the patient in a comfortable position.

2   Insert end of irrigation set into fluid pack and attach to infusion stand. Unclip the tubing and allow a small quantity of fluid to run through to expel the air.

3   Attach urine drainage bag to the **outlet end** of the three-way urethral catheter or to the urethral catheter.

4   Fix free end of the irrigation set to the **inlet** of the three-way urethral catheter or to the suprapubic

catheter. Undo the clip and allow the fluid to flow into the urinary bladder at a steady rate.

5   When the urine drainage bag is full, open outlet valve and collect returned fluid into a measuring container. Note the contents of the returned fluid.

6   Change irrigation fluid packs as necessary.

7   Record amount of irrigation fluid used and the amount of fluid returned via the urine drainage bag on the appropriate chart.

NOTE. **Urinary output** is estimated by subtracting the amount of irrigation fluid from the total fluid returned.

Observations and reporting

Note the presence of abnormalities in the returned fluid and report the result to the nurse in charge.

3.29
Gastric intubation

Gastric intubation is the passage of a tube into the stomach by one of the following routes:
    via the nose—the nasogastric route
    via the mouth—the orogastric route
A tube may also be inserted into the stomach through the anterior abdominal wall—gastrostomy. This is carried out by a surgeon in the operating theatre.

The passage of a nasogastric or orogastric tube may be used to:

1   Aspirate the stomach contents prior to, or following major oesophageal and abdominal operations.

2   Aspirate specimens of gastric juice for gastric function tests, e.g. pentagastrin test meal.

3   Aspirate the stomach contents in severe or prolonged vomiting, e.g. intestinal obstruction, severe haematemesis.

4   Facilitate tube feeding, e.g. in prolonged unconsciousness.

5   Wash out the stomach in pyloric stenosis or in certain forms of poison ingestion.

6   Aspirate gastric contents for cytological examination.

Dangers associated with gastric intubation
The tube may be passed into the respiratory tract. Any area with which the tube comes into contact may be damaged.

3

Routes
The **nasogastric route** is commonly used, except when passing larger stomach tubes. Difficulty is sometimes experienced when passing the tube if there is an **obstruction in the nostril,** e.g. nasal septal deviation, in which case the other nostril is used. **Always** check the nares to see which is the most patent. Occasionally the presence of a tube in the nose may deprive the patient of an adequate airway and therefore **must not** be used.

There is a danger that tubes passed via **the orogastric route** may be bitten through by some patients, e.g. semicomatosed or epileptic patients.

Therefore, if possible, the nasogastric route is used in these instances.

Equipment
A tray with the following:

Naso- or orogastric tube of suitable type. Usually 14 FG to 16 FG for an adult.

A gallipot of water (as a lubricant)

Box of tissues

Litmus (pH) papers

10 or 20 ml syringe in a disposable tray

Cotton buds and gallipot (if required to clean nares)

Measuring jug

Spigot

Tube retaining device or adhesive tape

Disposable sheet (towel) for protection of the patient

Disposal bag

Vomit bag

Denture carton (if required)

Preparation of the patient
Explain the procedure to the patient and gain his/her cooperation. Afford reassurance. Place the patient in a comfortable position sitting up well supported by pillows, if possible.

Procedure
1   Ensure privacy and arrange the protective towel over the patient's shoulders and chest.
2   Wash hands.

Nasogastric route. (a) Ensure the patient's nostrils are clean and remove his/her denture/s, if any, and place them in the denture carton.
(b) Check the nares and select the most patent for passage of the tube.
(c) Moisten the nasogastric tube with water, tilt the patient's head and gently ease the tube backwards along the floor of the nose.
(d) Instruct the patient to swallow while the tube is being passed and to breathe through the mouth. Sips of water may be given to aid the passage of the tube, if this is permitted. Pass the tube to a distance equal to length from patient's nose to his xiphisternum, measured when he is sitting upright.

Orogastric route. As per nasogastric procedure only in this instance the tube is passed via the mouth and not via the nose. When passing the tube over the patient's tongue **avoid** touching the uvula or any part of the soft palate.

Test to confirm the tube is in the stomach. The syringe is attached to the tube and a few millilitres of secretions are aspirated and placed in a gallipot. The secretions are tested for acidity with the litmus (pH) paper. A positive test usually indicates that the tube is in the stomach.

AND/OR

The free end of the tube is placed in a bowl of water. If there is *no distinct rhythmical bubbling* in the water, it is fairly safe to assume that the tube **is in the alimentary tract** and not the respiratory tract.

AND/OR

Two or three millilitres of air injected into the tube with the syringe and at the same time a stethoscope is placed over the patient's epigastrum. If the tube is in the stomach the injected air will be heard to 'gurgle' as it enters the stomach.

3   Once the tube is in the stomach it's free end is spigotted and secured comfortably to the patient's face, e.g. with a 'tube retainer'.

4   Any further procedures such as *gastric aspiration* (see Procedure 3.30) or *tube feeding* (see Procedure 3.32) can now be commenced.

NOTE. If difficulty is experienced when passing the tube, seek help from senior nursing staff.

Continuing care of the patient

1   Check at intervals that the tube is still in position and ensure that the patient is as comfortable as possible.

2   Give mouth washes at 2 hourly intervals or total mouth care to those patients unable to have a mouth wash, e.g. the unconscious patient (see Procedure 1.14).

3   Ensure that the patient's nostril/s are kept clean and free from crusting.

4   Keep the retaining tape (tube retainer) clean and replace as necessary.

5   Long-term tubes should be replaced weekly or as per manufacturer's instructions depending on type of tube used.

Removal of the tube
The 'tube retainer' is gently released. The spigot is left in the free end of the tube and using tissues to hold the tube it is gently and firmly removed and discarded.

Paediatric nursing notes
To secure the tube to the face appropriate strapping supplied from the nostril to the ear.

Double layer of tube-gauze mitts are used to cover the fingers of infants to prevent them from pulling at the tube.

3.30
Gastric aspiration

Gastric aspiration is the removal of gastric secretions by *Intermittent* or *Continuous aspiration* by means of a nasogastric or orogastric tube, more rarely via a gastrostomy tube.

It is used to:

 obtain specimens of gastric juice for biochemical analysis or cytological study

 prevent accumulation of secretions in the stomach before and after major abdominal operations, and in severe vomiting

 empty the stomach of food contents before emergency anaesthesia

Intermittent gastric aspiration
Aspiration is carried out at intervals, i.e. the entire stomach contents are gently withdrawn periodically, e.g. half hourly, hourly or 2 hourly intervals.

Equipment
As for gastric intubation (Procedure 3.29) plus a fluid balance chart or special test card to record: a description of the aspirate, the times of aspiration and the amounts of aspirate obtained.

Preparation of the patient
As per Procedure 3.29.

Procedure
1   The tube is passed as described under Procedure 3.29 and once it is confirmed that the tube is in the

patient's stomach, the syringe is attached and the entire stomach contents are aspirated and the amount obtained recorded.

2   A mouth wash may be given and the patient is left comfortable.

3   The procedure may be repeated at half hourly, hourly or 2 hourly intervals.

Continuous gastric aspiration
The gastic contents are withdrawn continuously by means of an electric suction machine which is attached to the free end of the intragastric tube. All aspirate is collected in a glass jar incorporated in the machine. The jar is emptied periodically and the aspirate measured and charted. The jar is thoroughly cleaned before replacement on the machine. **Alternatively** syphonage may be instituted by the attachment of a drainage bag plus tubing to the free end of the intragastric tube. To achieve effective syphonage the drainage bag must be situated lower than the patient's stomach. Periodic syringe aspiration will ensure patency of the intragastric tube.

Continuing care of the patient
As per Procedure 3.29.

3.31
Gastric lavage

Gastric lavage is the washing out of the stomach. It is used to wash out of the stomach some poisons and certain medicines and in medical and preoperative treatment of pyloric stenosis.

Equipment
Trolley with:
Funnel, tubing and connections
Stomach tube of a suitable size (usually 22–36 FG in the adult)
Jug containing 3 to 4 litres of fluid, e.g. tap water, normal saline or sodium bicarbonate 1 in 160 (0.625%)
Small jug 0.5 to 1 litre size
Bowl of water (as a lubricant)
Litmus (pH) paper
Box of tissues
Waterproof protection for the bed and the floor
Bucket
Disposable cap for the patient's hair
Waterproof protection for the nurse(s)
Specimen jar
Suction machine
Vomit bowl
Disposal bag

Preparation of the patient
Explain the procedure to the patient and gain his/ her cooperation.
Place the patient in a comfortable position, either

sitting in a chair or in bed well supported with pillows or lying on his/her side.

Remove patient's denture(s) if required and ensure privacy.

Procedure

1   Protect the bed and floor with the waterproof sheeting. Place the bucket for the returned fluid on the floor.

2   Put on waterproof protection and cover the patient's hair with a disposable cap.

3   Wash hands.

4   Moisten the stomach tube with water and pass via the patient's mouth taking care not to touch the patient's uvula and soft palate when passing it over the tongue. Instruct the patient to swallow as the tube is being passed.

NOTE. Observe the patient's colour during the procedure. If he/she becomes cyanosed **immediately** withdraw the tube.

5   Check that the tube is in the stomach by either: placing the free end of the tube under water to ascertain it is not in the respiratory tract;

OR

by aspirating secretions with a large nozzled aspirating syringe and testing with litmus (pH) paper for acidity (see Procedure 3.29, tests to confirm the tube is in the stomach).

6   Connect up the apparatus (funnel, tubing and connections) to the free end of the stomach tube. Hold the funnel over the bucket to allow the escape of gas and stomach contents. This can be collected as a specimen.

NOTE. In **some cases** of poisoning aspirate stomach contents **before** commencing gastric lavage. Aspirate is kept as a specimen. A bladder syringe with a central nozzle can be used for aspiration.

7   Using the small jug pour 0.5 litre of fluid into the funnel and allow the fluid to run in evenly. **Before** the funnel is empty invert it over the bucket and syphon back the fluid.

8   Continue in this manner (item 7) until the fluid is clear.

9   Clamp and carefully remove the tube and make the patient comfortable.

10   Measure and record the amount and type of fluid administered and returned.

11   The specimen may be kept in the ward for inspection by the medical staff or sent on medical instructions to the laboratory with the appropriate form and details.

Aftercare of equipment

All disposable equipment is placed in the appropriate container.

All non-disposable equipment is thoroughly washed and cleaned and returned to appropriate storage units. The trolley is thoroughly cleaned.

Special nursing note

Gastric lavage of an unconscious patient is often done in accident and emergency units where it is the doctor's responsibility. An anaesthetist is usually present to intubate the trachea.

Suction apparatus should be available in **all** cases.

3.32
Tube Feeding

Tube feeding is the introduction of liquid into the stomach via a tube passed through the nose or the mouth or through an artificial opening, e.g. a gastrostomy.

It is used during prolonged unconsciousness and dysphagia and following surgical operations on the mouth, pharynx, larynx or oesophagus. It may be necessary for feeding premature or weakly babies who are unable to suck and for feeding severely depressed or anorexic patients.

Equipment
As for Gastric intubation (see Procedure 3.29) plus:
Funnel or 20–50 ml syringe barrel
Measuring jug containing the amount of feed to be given
Bowl of hot water (for warming the food **only**)
Measure containing 60 ml of water
Disposal bag

The feed
The aim is to give the patient all the essential nutrients. This can be achieved by giving:
    food reconstituted with milk or water
    liquidised diet suitable for the patient's needs
    pre-prepared food which can be reconstituted
The food should be warmed in a bowl of hot water before administration.
The average amount given per day for an adult is 8400–10 000 kJ in 2500–3000 ml of fluid.

3

Procedure

1 Explain the procedure to the patient and place him/her in a comfortable sitting position (if conscious). (If the tube is not in situ, pass it as per Procedure 3.29, Gastric intubation.)

2 Check that tube is in position by withdrawing a small amount of gastric contents with the syringe and testing with litmus (pH) paper for acidity.

3 The funnel or syringe barrel is attached to the end of the intragastric tube and 30 ml of water is run slowly through the tube holding the funnel or syringe barrel slightly above the patient's head.

4 The feed is then given slowly, ensuring that the funnel or syringe barrel never become empty. When the correct amount of feed has been given, a further 30 ml of water is run through to clear the tube.

5 The funnel or syringe barrel is removed and the intragastric tube spigotted or clipped and the tube secured or removed.

6 Oral hygiene is then carried out (see Procedures 1.13, and 1.14).

7 The patient is left comfortable and the amount of fluid given is recorded on the appropriate chart.

Aftercare of equipment

All non-disposable equipment is thoroughly washed and cleaned.

Special nursing notes

Observe that no vomiting occurs after a feed.

Passive or active resistance with reference to eating and taking of food and nourishment by a psychiatric patient may, in the best interests of the patient, necessitate him/her being placed on an Emergency Certificate by the Medical Staff (see Mental Health Act (Scotland) 1960).

3.33
Exploration and aspiration of the pleural cavity

Exploration and aspiration of the pleural cavity may be carried out as a diagnostic procedure to examine the pleural fluid and determine any micro-organisms present. It may also be carried out as a therapeutic measure to relieve dyspnoea and/or to introduce medicines into the pleural cavity.

Equipment

Basic trolley for sterile procedures (see Procedure 3.16) plus:

Local anaesthetic with syringe and needle

20 or 50 ml syringe

Two-way tap with a length of tubing attached to one of the arms

Aspirating needles of different sizes

Sterile bowl to collect aspirate

Measuring jug for aspirate

Specimen bottles

Collodion Nobecutane or Air Strip to seal the puncture

Sterile gloves

Recent chest X-rays at hand

If a medicine is to be introduced into the pleural cavity:

Syringe, needles and the prescribed medicine

Prescription and medicine recording sheets

3

Preparation of the patient
1   Ensure that the procedure is explained to the patient.
2   A back fastening gown is put on the patient.
3   The patient sits up with his/her arms extended over a bed table with a pillow on which to rest his/her head. If able to, the patient may sit on the side of the bed with his/her feet supported on a stool.
4   Instruct the patient to indicate if he/she feels pain or wants to cough during the course of the procedure.

Procedure
1   Take trolley to the bedside and ensure privacy.
2   Mask and wash hands. Assist the doctor.
3   The doctor cleans the patient's skin, injects the local anaesthetic and then inserts the aspirating needle attached to the two-way tap. The nurse should be ready with the specimen bottles. The remainder of the fluid is collected into the sterile bowl and then measured.
4   The doctor withdraws the aspirating needle and applies a collodion dressing of Nobecutane or an Air Strip to seal the puncture.
5   Measure the fluid, noting the colour and record the amount obtained on the patient's fluid balance chart.
6   Specimens labelled and sent with the appropriate forms to the laboratory.
7   Clear away equipment, leave the patient comfortable and unscreen the bed.
   NOTE. Normally after the procedure a post-aspiration chest X-ray is carried out.

Observations
Aspiration of the pleural cavity can occasionally cause shock, so it is important during the procedure

to observe the patient's colour and respiration rate. After the procedure the patient is observed and the pulse is recorded half-hourly or as per medical instructions.

Aftercare of equipment
As per Procedure 3.16.

3.34
Lumbar puncture

A lumbar puncture is performed to:
  obtain a specimen of cerebrospinal fluid for ex-
    amination
  ascertain the pressure of cerebrospinal fluid
  remove some cerebrospinal fluid prior to the in-
    troduction of medicines or radio-opaque fluid
    for diagnostic purposes.
  The site of the puncture is between the third and
    fourth or fourth and fifth lumbar vertebrae.

Equipment
Basic trolley for sterile procedures (Procedure 3.16)
plus:
Local anaesthetic with syringe and needles
Two-way adaptor
Lumbar puncture needles
Disposable manometer set
Sterile gloves
Sterile drapes
Collodion Nobecutane or Air Strip to seal puncture
Packet with 3 sterile universal containers plus
  glucose estimation bottle
If a medicine is to be introduced:
  syringe, needles and the prescribed medicine
  prescription and medicine recording sheets

Preparation of the patient
1   Ensure that the procedure has been explained to
the patient.
2   Place the patient in the lateral position near the

edge of the bed. The neck and shoulders should be flexed and the knees drawn up to the chest. A pillow may be left under his/her head. The assistance of a second nurse may be required to maintain this position.

3   Expose the patient's lumbar region only.

Procedure

1   Take the trolley to the bedside and ensure privacy.

2   Mask and wash hands. Assist the doctor.

3   The doctor cleans the patient's skin and injects the local anaesthetic and surrounds the area with sterile drapes. He/she then inserts the lumbar puncture needle, removes the stillete and attaches the two-way tap. A manometer reading (80–150 mm fluid) may then be taken. A specimen of cerebrospinal fluid is then collected.

4   The nurse may be asked to compress the jugular veins on either side of the patient's neck—Queckenstedt's Test.

5   The nurse should be prepared to collect further specimens of cerebrospinal fluid.

6   The doctor withdraws the lumbar puncture needle and applies a collodion dressing, Nobecutane or Air Strip to seal the puncture.

7   The doctor records the colour and pressures of the cerebrospinal fluid.

8   Specimens labelled and sent with appropriate forms to the laboratory.

9   The patient is advised to lie flat for 4 to 6 hours to prevent headache. The foot of the bed may be elevated.

10   Clear away equipment, leave the patient comfortable and unscreen the bed.

Observations
A lumbar puncture may occasionally cause shock, so it is important during the procedure to observe the patient's colour and respiration rate. After the procedure the patient is observed and the pulse is recorded as per medical instructions.

Aftercare of equipment
As per Procedure 3.16.

3.35
Cisternal puncture

A cisternal puncture is an alternative method to the lumbar puncture for obtaining cerebrospinal fluid. It is only used in special cases.

The equipment required for a cisternal puncture is similar to that required for Procedure 3.34, Lumbar puncture, except that a special needle with its shaft marked off in centimetres is used.

The site of the puncture is at the junction of the skull and spine and the skin over this area may require to be shaved prior to commencement of the procedure.

3.36
Abdominal paracentesis

Abdominal paracentesis is the withdrawal of fluid from the peritoneal cavity. Free fluid in the peritoneal cavity is called *Ascites*. Causes of this condition are:

 right-sided heart failure

 cirrhosis of the liver

 malignant conditions with metastases in the peritoneal cavity

An abdominal paracentesis is carried out as a diagnostic measure to ascertain the presence and type of cells or micro-organisms present in the peritoneal fluid.

As a therapeutic measure it is used to:

 relieve pressure on abdominal and thoracic organs, so relieve the dyspnoea in right-sided heart failure

 introduce medicines into the peritoneal cavity, e.g. cytotoxic agents in malignant disease

Dangers associated with abdominal paracentesis

Puncture of an abdominal organ

Introduction of infection

Collapse due to sudden release of fluid in peritoneal cavity

Puncture of the bladder

Equipment

Basic trolley for sterile procedures (see Procedure 3.16) plus:

Local anaesthetic with syringe and needles

Trocar and cannula
Medicut with recipient set
Sterile tubing to fit the cannula
Disposable scalpel
Sterile gloves
Disposable drainage bag with bottom outlet
Tube clip (gate clip)
Specimen bottle
Abdominal binder

Preparation of the patient

1   Ensure that the procedure is explained to the patient.
2   It is **essential** that the patient's urinary bladder is empty so that there is no danger of puncture. It may be necessary for urinary catheterisation to be carried out prior to commencement of the procedure.
3   Place the patient in a comfortable position, either recumbent or well supported with pillows.
4   Place the abdominal binder in position.

Procedure

1   Take the trolley to the bedside and ensure privacy.
2   Mask and wash hands. Assist the doctor.
3   The doctor cleans the patient's skin and injects the local anaesthetic and surrounds the area with sterile drapes. He/she then inserts the trocar and cannula (Medicut), removes the trocar and attaches the tubing to the cannula (recipient set). If a specimen of the peritoneal fluid is required for laboratory test, it is usually collected at this stage.
4   The end of the tubing is connected to the drainage bag.
5   The tube clip (gate clip) is applied to the tubing

and adjusted so that the peritoneal fluid flows at the desired rate. (The control of the recipient set serves the same purpose.)

6   The cannula (Medicut) is kept in position with strapping and a small sterile dressing.

7   The abdominal binder is applied.

8   Specimen is labelled and sent with the appropriate form to the laboratory.

9   Clear away equipment, leave the patient comfortable and unscreen the bed.

Continuing care of the patient

1   The abdominal binder is adjusted at intervals to maintain support.

2   Check puncture wound for leakage or signs of inflammation.

3   Empty drainage bag at intervals, as necessary.

4   The amount and colour of the peritoneal fluid is recorded on the fluid balance chart.

5   When the peritoneal fluid has stopped draining the cannula (Medicut) is removed under septic technique and a sterile dressing applied to the puncture site. The binder is adjusted.

Aftercare of equipment

As per Procedure 3.16.

3.37
Removal of fluid from oedematous subcutaneous tissues of the legs

3

In certain cases where there is no real reduction in oedema after other treatments. The following methods are sometimes prescribed to remove fluid from oedematous subcutaneous tissues of the legs.

There are two methods (both are now seldom used):
Southey's tubes
Acupuncture

Southey's tubes
Southey's tubes consist of a set of 4 to 6 cannulae of different lengths with one trocar. Lengths of fine tubing and the set are supplied.

The limbs are usually in the dependent position before commencement of the treatment,—a special cardiac bed. The skin is cleansed, anaesthetised and each cannula is introduced by using the trocar. The cannulae are kept in position by narrow adhesive tape. The ends of the tubing are inserted into a drainage receptacle. The cannulae may be left in situ for 24 hours or more and during this time the drained fluid is measured and recorded. After the treatment is complete a sterile dressing is applied and renewed as required.

Acupuncture (Scarification)
Acupuncture consists of making a number of small

incisions, e.g. with a scalpel or cutting needle, and the fluid is allowed to drain into sterile dressings. Adequate protection of the bed must be ensured before commencement of the procedure.

3

3.38
Stoma care

Early preparation of the patient

Admission. As the physical and mental pre-operative preparation is most important in a stoma operation the patient is usually admitted 3 to 5 days prior to the operation.

The surgeon will inform the patient about the operation and will usually mark the area where he/she hopes to construct the stoma. If possible a stoma-therapist should visit the patient on admission to discuss stoma appliances and care and to show the appliances available.

Stoma appliance. Prior to the operation the patient wears a stoma appliance over the possible stoma site in order to get accustomed to the weight and feel of the bag. The bag of the urinary conduit patient should contain 100 ml water. The bag of the ileostomy/colostomy patient should contain a two-pence piece.

The position of the bag may be altered if there is the possibility of leakage due to skin folds or pressure and discomfort from skirt/trouser waist band.

Allergic reactions. Possible allergic reactions are detected early by the application to the patient's skin of adhesive tapes, karya gum, stomahesive, other adhesives and sprays. The wearing of the stoma appliance may also show up any allergic reaction.

Booklets. There are excellent booklets which explain in simple language every aspect of life with a stoma. These should be made available for the patient.

Immediate preoperative preparation. Immediate preoperative preparation is carried out as for abdominal rectal surgery.

3

3.39
Postoperative stoma care

3

Postoperative stoma care is carried out to cleanse the skin and observe the stoma.

Equipment
Trolley with:
Gauze swabs in a receiver
Bowl
Aqueous solution for wound cleaning
Suitable stoma appliance, e.g. Holister bag
Skin protector, e.g. Skin gel (if required)
Stomahesive or similar adhesive (if required)
Disposal bag
  NOTE. This is not a sterile procedure but all care **must** be taken to prevent unnecessary contamination.

Preparation of the patient
Explain the procedure fully to the patient as he/she will be very apprehensive especially in the instance of the first removal of the stoma appliance.

Procedure
1   Take the trolley to the bedside and ensure privacy.
2   Place the patient in a comfortable position. Wash hands.
3   Gently remove the used stoma appliance and discard.

3

4 Using swabs and the recommended wound cleansing solution carefully and gently cleanse the peristomal skin (skin surrounding the stoma). Using separate swabs and the wound solution cleanse the stoma in a similar manner. Dry the peristomal skin thoroughly.

5 Inspect the stoma for peristalsis, size and colour. Inspect the peristomal skin and if it is red or excoriated report this to the nurse in charge.

NOTE. While the stoma appliance is off the patient should be encouraged to look at the stoma. A hand-mirror can be used for this purpose.

6 If the peristomal skin is red a skin protector is used before adhering the stoma appliance, e.g. Skin gel or Dow Corning adhesive spray.

7 Ensure that the peristomal skin is thoroughly dry and apply the stoma appliance from below adhering the flange from the bottom first, then the side and finally the top. Check that there are no folds or creases in the adhesive flange and ensure that it is securely in position.

NOTE. **Always** allow 4 mm between the stoma and the flange of the appliance.

The patient should be observing the nurse throughout the procedure knowing that in the future he/she will be caring for the stoma. It is important, therefore to explain to the patient everything that is being done and the reasons for doing same.

8 Clear away equipment, leave the patient comfortable and unscreen the bed.

Aftercare of equipment
Disposal bag and its contents placed in appropriate container.

The trolley is thoroughly cleaned with detergent and hot water and/or recommended disinfectant.

Observations and reporting
Inspect the stoma for peristalsis, size and colour. Note the condition of the peristomal skin. Report to the nurse in charge.

3.40
Continuing stoma care

3

Continuing stoma care will allow cleansing of the stoma and ensure healthy peristomal skin.

The long-term care of stoma differs from the immediate postoperative in that Savlon (centrimide chlorhexidine gluconate) or similar solutions **are not used** as skin irritation may develop if used over a long period of time.

Equipment
As for Procedure 3.39 but excluding the wound cleaning lotion, plus:
Mild soap in a dish
Bowl of warm water (33–35°C)
Absorbent tissues

Preparation of the patient
Explain the procedure to the patient and encourage him/her to participate.

Procedure
1   As per Procedure 3.39 with the exception of cleansing with lotion. In this instance the peristomal skin and the stoma are thoroughly but gently washed with mild soap using absorbent tissues.
2   A suitable belt and a disposable stoma bag cover may be applied, if desired.

Aftercare of equipment
As per Procedure 3.39.

Observations and reporting
As per Procedure 3.39.

3.41
Special biopsies

A biopsy is the removal of a small specimen of tissue from a body organ in which disease is suspected, in order that pathological examination can be undertaken.

An explanation of the procedure is given to the patient and written consent of the patient is obtained.

In children biopsies are normally carried out under a general anaesthetic. See Procedure 8.13 for a jejunal biopsy using a Crosby capsule.

It is normal practice for biopsies to be performed in a designated treatment area.

3.42
Needle biopsy of the liver (using the intercostal route)

3

Needle biopsy of the liver is the removal of a minute piece of liver tissue for pathological examination.

Prior to procedure
The patient's blood should be typed and cross matched. Clotting studies are carried out.
The patient may be prescribed sedation 30 to 60 minutes before the procedure. See Procedure 3.41.

Equipment
Basic trolley for sterile procedures (see Procedure 3.16) plus:
Liver biopsy needle (e.g. *Menghini*)
20 ml syringe
Local anaesthetic with syringe and needles
Disposable scalpel
Sterile gloves
Bottle of normal saline
Small adhesive dressing
Specimen jar with preservative

Preparation of the patient
The procedure is explained to the patient and he/she is assisted into a supine position, slightly rotated so that the right shoulder is a little more anterior than the left. His/her head is turned to the left and supported by a pillow.

3

Procedure

1   Take the trolley to the bedside and ensure privacy.

2   Mask and wash hands. Assist the doctor.

3   The doctor cleans the patient's skin and injects the rib space with local anaesthetic.

   NOTE. The patient is asked to breathe in and then breathe out as far as possible—this ensures the diaphragm is as high as possible.

4   The doctor then inserts the biopsy needle, attached to the 20 ml syringe containing 3 ml of normal saline. The patient is then asked to hold his breath in full expiration and the doctor withdraws the needle and the syringe which should contain the liver specimen.

5   A small adhesive dressing is applied over the puncture site.

6   The specimen is placed in the specimen jar which is clearly labelled and sent with the appropriate form to the laboratory.

   NOTE. The patient is asked to lie on his/her right side for 2 hours and to remain in bed for 24 hours.

7   Clear away the equipment, leave the patient comfortable and unscreen the bed.

Aftercare and observation of the patient

See Note after item 6 of Procedure.

The patient's pulse and blood pressure are recorded for 24 hours—every 15 minutes for the first 2 hours following the procedure. Report if tachycardia or any change in the quality of the pulse occurs to the nurse in charge. Report change in blood pressure.

An analgesic may be prescribed by the doctor if the patient complains of shoulder-tip pain (referred pain).

Aftercare of equipment
As per Procedure 3.16.

Complications
Haemorrhage due to rupture of the liver.
Biliary peritonitis due to rupture of the biliary system.

3.43
Renal biopsy

3

Renal biopsy is the removal of a minute piece of kidney for pathological examination. It may possibly be carried out in the X-ray department.

Prior to the procedure
The patient will have had an intravenous pyelography.
See Procedure 3.41.

Equipment
Basic trolley for sterile procedures (see Procedure 3.16) plus:
Renal exploration needle
Renal biopsy needle
20 ml syringe
Local anaesthetic with syringe and needles
Disposable scalpel
Sterile gloves
Strapping
Specimen jar
Sandbag
X-rays (intravenous pyelography)

Preparation of the patient
The procedure is explained to the patient and he/she is assisted into the prone position with the sandbag placed under the abdomen. The area of the lumbar region is marked by the doctor.

Procedure
1   Take the trolley to the bedside and ensure privacy.

3

2   Check the patient's position.

3   Mask and wash hands. Assist the doctor.

4   The doctor cleans the patient's skin and injects the area with local anaesthetic.

5   The doctor then inserts the renal exploration needle and explores the area to confirm the kidney position. The exploration needle is withdrawn and the renal biopsy needle inserted. The doctor withdraws the biopsy needle and the syringe and the kidney specimen is placed in the specimen jar.

6   A **very firm dressing** is then applied over the puncture site.

NOTE. The patient is asked to lie in the prone position for 1 hour and to remain in bed for 24 hours.

7   The specimen jar which is clearly labelled is sent with the appropriate form to the laboratory.

8   Clear away equipment, leave the patient comfortable and unscreen the bed.

Aftercare and observation of the patient

1   See Note after item 6 of Procedure.

2   The patient's blood pressure and pulse rate are recorded every 30 minutes for 24 hours. Urinary output is charted and urine tested for the presence of blood (haematuria).

3   Complaint of lumbar or shoulder region pain by the patient should be reported **immediately** to the nurse in charge.

Aftercare of equipment
As per Procedure 3.16.

Complications
Difficulty in passing urine.
Bleeding from the biopsy puncture site.

3.44
Marrow biopsy (puncture)

3

Marrow biopsy is the removal of a specimen of red
  bone marrow for pathological examination.

Examination of the red bone marrow helps in the
  diagnosis of certain blood conditions.

The area selected for the biopsy is the sternum or
  the iliac crest of the pelvis.

Prior to procedure
See Procedure 3.41.

The patient may be prescribed sedation 30 minutes
before the procedure.

The sternal area may require to be shaved.

Equipment
Basic trolley for sterile procedures (see Procedure
3.16) plus:

*Sternal puncture needle (Salah's needle or trocar
and cannula)

*20 ml syringe

*Glass slides

Local anaesthetic with syringe and needles

Sterile gloves

Collodion or Nobecutane to seal the puncture

Disposable drapes

Preparation of the patient
The procedure is explained to the patient and he/

---

* These are usually brought from the laboratory by the doctor
carrying out the procedure or the laboratory technician.

she is assisted into the recumbent position. A pillow may, in addition, be placed under the shoulders.

Procedure

1 Take the trolley to the bedside and ensure privacy.
2 Check the patient's position.
3 Mask and wash hands. Assist the doctor.
4 The doctor cleans the patient's skin, places drapes in position and injects the area with local anaesthetic.
5 The doctor inserts the sternal puncture needle to a pre-determined depth only, attaches the syringe and withdraws a specimen of red bone marrow.
6 The needle is withdrawn and the puncture is sealed with collodion or Nobecutane. A small dressing is applied.
7 The doctor or technician places some of the red bone marrow specimen on the glass slides.
8 Clear away equipment, leave the patient comfortable and unscreen the bed.

Nursing note
The patient's eyes may be covered during the procedure if required.

Aftercare of patient

The puncture site is observed for bleeding and the patient should remain in bed for at least 2 hours.

Aftercare of equipment

As per Procedure 3.16 with the exception that the sternal puncture needle (trocar and cannula) is returned to the laboratory.

3.45
Pleural biopsy

3

Pleural biopsy is the removal of a minute piece of pleura for pathological examination.

The procedure is **only** done when fluid is present between the layers of the pleura as otherwise there is danger to the underlying lung.

Prior to the procedure
See Procedure 3.41.
The patient will have had a chest x-ray.

Equipment
Basic trolley for sterile procedures (Procedure 3.16) plus:
Abram's pleural biopsy needle
20 ml syringe
Disposable scalpel
Local anaesthetic with syringe and needles
Suturing material
Sterile gloves
Specimen jar with preservative
Recent chest x-rays at hand

Preparation of the patient
As per Procedure 3.33, Exploration and aspiration of the pleural cavity.

Procedure
1   Take the trolley to the bedside and ensure privacy.
2   Mask and wash hands. Assist the doctor.

3   The doctor cleans the patient's skin, injects the area with local anaesthetic and then makes a small incision with the scalpel blade. The biopsy needle is attached to the syringe and the doctor introduces the needle, with a rotating movement, into the selected intercostal space. The biopsy needle is withdrawn and the specimen of pleura is placed in the specimen jar.

4   The doctor closes the tract with a single suture and a small dressing is applied.

5   The specimen jar which is clearly labelled is sent with the appropriate form to the laboratory.

NOTE. The patient is asked to remain in bed for 5 to 6 hours.

6   Clear away equipment, leave the patient comfortable and unscreen the bed.

NOTE. Normally after the procedure a post pleural biopsy chest x-ray is carried out.

Aftercare and observation of the patient
1   See Note after item 5 of Procedure.

2   Note the quality of the patient's breathing for 5 to 6 hours.

3   The patient's blood pressure and pulse rate are recorded every 30 minutes until settled, then every 2 hours thereafter or as per medical instructions.

4   An analgesic may be prescribed by the doctor if the patient complains of pain.

Aftercare of equipment
As per Procedure 3.16.

Complication
During the procedure it is most important **not** to introduce air into the pleural cavity. Otherwise this will cause a *pneumothorax* with signs of increasing dyspnoea.

3.46
Suction biopsy of the small intestine using a Crosby capsule

Suction biopsy of the small intestine is the removal, using a Crosby capsule, of a minute piece of the small intestine for pathological examination.

A **Crosby capsule** is a long thin x-ray opaque tube with a luer fitting at one end (to which a syringe can be attached) and a small metal capsule incorporating a guillotine device at the other end.

The procedure is carried out by a doctor in the x-ray department.

Prior to the procedure
See Procedure 3.41.
The patient is fasted overnight and an explanation of the procedure is given.

Equipment
Crosby capsule
20 ml syringe
Gauze swabs
Gallipot
Water for lubrication
Adhesive tape
Universal container

Preparation of the patient
An explanation of the procedure is again given to the patient and he/she is placed in the sitting up position.

Procedure

1   The doctor lubricates the tube and places the capsule on the back of the patient's tongue and asks him/her to swallow.

2   Once the capsule has entered the stomach, the patient is asked to lie down on his/her right side. (This assists the capsule to move, by peristalsis, down the gastrointestinal tract.)

3   The free end of the tube is fixed to the patient's gown or face with adhesive tape.

4   The position of the capsule is checked by x-ray and screening before the biopsy is taken.

5   The doctor attaches the syringe to the luer end of the tube and introduces air. He/she will then pull the syringe piston up several times to create a vacuum within the tube and cause the lining of the small intestine to be pulled into the side of the capsule.

6   The syringe piston is finally drawn up and released sharply. (This causes activation of the guillotine device within the capsule and a small piece of the intestine wall is drawn into the tube.)

7   The tube is gently and carefully removed and the specimen from the Crosby capsule is taken in universal container to the laboratory as soon as possible with the appropriate form.

8   On return to the ward the patient is made comfortable and is given a mouthwash.

Aftercare of patient

1   The patient's pulse and respiration rates are recorded hourly or as per medical instruction.

2   The patient is observed for bleeding.

Aftercare of the Crosby capsule

The tube and the capsule are cleaned with clean

water and left immersed in appropriate disinfectant solution. It is then carefully dried and returned to its box.

3.47
Peritoneal dialysis

Peritoneal dialysis accomplishes similar functions and operates on the same principles of diffusion and osmosis as haemodialysis. In this instance, the peritoneum is the semipermeable membrane.

It is used in acute and chronic renal failure, intractable oedema and severe anaemia and other electrolyte disturbances.

Equipment for manual dialysis
(A machine may also be used)
Basic trolley for sterile procedures (see Procedure 3.16) plus:
A box containing instruments, connecting lines, suturing material, sterile gowns
Dialysing fluid and apparatus to warm it to 40°C
Prescribed medicines
Drainage bag and tap effluent container

Preparation of the patient
1   The abdomen is shaved and prepared.
2   Vital signs such as temperature, pulse and respiration and blood pressure are recorded. Weight must also be recorded.
3   The urinary bladder should be emptied to prevent puncture with the trocar.
   NOTE. Specific orders regarding fluid removal, replacement and medicine administration should be written out by the doctor and when necessary administered by him.

Procedure

The setting up of peritoneal dialysis is done by the doctor. The nurse may assist.

Continuing nursing care

Accurate fluid intake and output records to assess volume depletion or overload.

Frequent checking of the patient's vital signs, weight, general condition, and effluent.

Attention to the patient's mouth, pressure areas and movement of limbs.

The patient's diet is not restricted during dialysis and he/she should be encouraged to eat a **normal diet**.

Complications

1   Incomplete recovery of fluid with each exchange. The fluid removed should be at least equal to or exceed the amount of fluid inserted.

NOTE. If there is retention of fluid (*positive balance*) turning the patient from side to side, elevating the head of the bed or gently massaging the patient's abdomen can help. Alternatively the patient may be encouraged to cough vigorously. If these measures fail the **doctor must be informed**.

2   Pain—the patient may feel some abdominal discomfort during the procedure. The doctor may prescribe a mild analgesic.

3   Peritonitis.

NOTE. First and last specimens of fluid are sent with appropriate forms to the laboratory.

3.48
Underwater seal pleural drainage

Underwater seal pleural drainage is used to remove blood, air, pus or serous fluid from the pleural cavity in thoracotomy, chest injury or pneumothorax.

Equipment
Basic trolley for sterile procedures (see Procedure 3.16) plus:
*Large Winchester bottle (containing 500 ml of sterile water or normal saline)·
*Rubber cork pierced by short and long glass or rigid plastic tubes
Trocar and cannula (may be used)
Intercostal tubing and introducer
2 pairs of tubing clamps in a receiver
Disposable scalpel
Local anaesthetic with syringe and needles
Suturing material
Sterile gloves
Specimen jar
Suction machine
Recent chest x-rays

Preparation of equipment
Large Winchester bottle containing 500 ml of sterile water or normal saline. The level of the fluid in the bottle is marked with strapping or preferably a graduated bottle may be used.

* These may be available as a pack

Two-holed rubber cork is pierced by a short and a long glass or rigid plastic tubes. The long tube is submerged in the fluid for 2–3 cm but **must not touch** the bottom of the bottle. The short tube acts as an escape route for air. A length of tubing is connected to the top end of the underwater tubing (the long tube) and to a connector. The connector is then joined to the patient's intercostal drainage tube. The whole tubing **must be** of sufficient length to allow the patient ease of movement in bed. (See Fig. 11.)

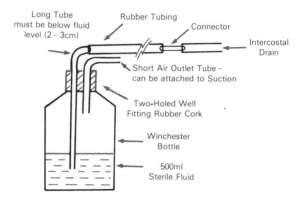

Fig. 11 Prepared equipment for underwater seal pleural drainage.

Preparation of the patient
The procedure is carefully explained to the patient and his/her cooperation is obtained.

Procedure
1 Take the trolley to the bedside and ensure privacy.
2 Mask and wash hands. Assist the doctor.

3 (Box with number 3)

3 The usual site for insertion of the intercostal tube is laterally between the fifth and sixth ribs. In order to achieve maximum separation of the intercostal space at the site for insertion of the intercostal tube the patient is positioned leaning over a bed table supported by pillows. The arm on the side of insertion of the tube **must be placed forward** and supported by a nurse who also observes the patient's colour, pulse and respiration rates during the procedure.

4 The doctor cleans the patient's skin, places drapes in position and injects the area with local anaesthetic. He/she then makes a small incision through the skin and muscle of the intercostal space with the scalpel. The doctor using the introducer inserts the intercostal tubing and retains it in position by a purse string suture.

5 The nurse must have the connecting tube end of the assembled underwater seal apparatus ready to connect immediately to the intercostal tube once the introducer is removed.

NOTE. The intercostal tube **must be clamped** with the **two pairs** of tubing clamps until all connections of the apparatus are sealed. Strapping can be applied to the joints to ensure this.

6 The tubing clamps are removed and the functioning of the apparatus is checked by noting if oscillations of fluid are occurring in the long tube (underwater tube) in rhythm with the patient's respiration rate. (The short air outlet tube is connected up to a suction machine if suction is used.)

7 A dressing is applied to the wound.

8 Clear away equipment, leave the patient comfortable and unscreen the bed. Re-check the functioning of the apparatus.

Special nursing notes

1   All connections of the underwater seal apparatus **must be secure**. (See Note after item 5 of Procedure.)

2   Ensure that the patient is **not compressing or kinking** any part of the drainage system.

3   Ensure that the tubing is of sufficient length to allow easy movement of the patient in bed.

4   The Winchester bottle **must always remain below the level of the patient's chest** either by standing the bottle in a container on the floor or attached to the side of the patient's bed.

NOTE. **All** members of staff must be instructed **never** to move the bottle above the level of the bed unless the drainage tube is firmly clamped with the **two pairs** of clamps.

5   If suction is used **check** that the machine maintains the pressure set by the doctor.

6   The rate and quantity of drainage is observed and the amount of the latter is recorded on the appropriate chart.

NOTE. A Heimlich valve may be used instead of the underwater seal equipment. The valve is attached to a drainage bag.

Aftercare of equipment
As per Procedure 3.16.

Changing a bottle
To change a bottle **securely clamp off** the intercostal drain with the **two clamps**, disconnect tubing at the connection and put used apparatus to the side.

Connect fresh tubing and carry out items 1 to 4 inclusive of Special nursing notes and if in order remove the clamps and note if the oscillations of

fluid in the underwater tube (long tube) are occurring in rhythm with the patient's respiration rate.

Record the amount of drainage on the appropriate
chart and attend to the used apparatus.

3

3.49
Underwater seal pleural drainage—removal of the intercostal drain

3

Prior to the procedure
The patient may be prescribed an analgesic 30 minutes before the procedure.

Equipment
Basic trolley for sterile procedure (see Procedure 3.16) plus:
Stitch scissors
Tulle gras
Waterproof strapping
Bacteriological swab and appropriate form
   NOTE. If a retaining purse string suture was omitted on the introduction of the intercostal tube, additional equipment for local anaesthetic and suturing (see Procedure 3.48, page 175) are required in order that the doctor may introduce a purse string suture prior to removal of the tube.

Preparation of the patient
The procedure is explained to the patient and his cooperation gained.

Procedure
This would be carried out by a doctor and a nurse, both functioning as **dressers**. If no suturing required, two nurses (one of whom must be an experienced trained nurse) may undertake the procedure.
1   Take the trolley to the bedside and ensure privacy.
2   Mask and wash hands.
3   **Securely clamp off** the intercostal drain with the two tubing clamps, disconnect tubing at the

connection and put used apparatus to one side.

4 Prepare appropriate lengths of waterproof strapping.

5 Wash hands.

6 Both **dressers** prepare the dressing. The nurse carefully removes the old dressing and cleans the wound area while the doctor prepares a dressing with tulle gras, a quantity of gauze swabs and waterproof strapping.

NOTES. At this point in the procedure, the doctor may introduce a purse string suture, if required.

If the intercostal tube is held in position by a purse string suture this will be visible by two long ends.

The intercostal tube should be gently and slightly rotated before removal.

7 The intercostal tube is removed by instructing the patient to take a deep breath and hold it. When he does this, nurse quickly but gently pulls out the intercostal drain and covers the opening with the prepared dressing, while the doctor **immediately** securely ties off the suture. The patient is then instructed to breathe freely once the tube has been removed. It is often the practice to take a bacteriological swab from the proximal end of the intercostal tube once the tube has been removed. Care must be taken to avoid contamination of the tube until the swab has been taken.

8 A chest x-ray is then carried out.

9 Clear away equipment, leave the patient comfortable and unscreen the bed.

10 The amount of drainage in the Winchester bottle is recorded on the appropriate chart.

Aftercare of equipment

As per Procedure 3.16 plus attention to the underwater seal apparatus.

3.50
The use and care of Redivac drains

3

The purpose of a drain is to withdraw any exudate or fluid from a cavity after a surgical operation.

1   Continuous vacuum in the Redivac bottle **must be maintained**. This is ensured by observing that the antennae are wide apart. (These are the two rubber horns which protrude through the top of the stopper of the bottle.)

2   The Redivac bottle should be renewed at least once per day or as necessary. The drainage tube from the wound **must be securely clamped off** when the bottle is being changed.

3   Ensure that there is no kinking or compression of the drainage tube.

4   The drainage is measured and recorded accurately on the appropriate chart. A specimen may be taken at this stage and sent to the laboratory with the appropriate form.

5   Sterile bottles are vacuumed in the ward using mechanical suction.

6   The bottle is attached to the side of the bed using a small metal clip.

7   Used bottles are washed and rinsed.

3.51
Monitor (chest lead) toilet

Monitor toilet is the special nursing care required for the patient who is attached to a cardiac oscilloscope. It is performed in order to:
   give the best possible electrocardiogram picture while ensuring patient comfort
   clean and maintain the electrodes
   ensure that no skin reaction has occurred

Equipment
Bowl of warm water (33–35°C)
Packet of tissues/clean swabs
Replacement electrodes or adhesive discs
Electrode cream
Roll of adhesive tape 2.5 cm wide if required
Disposal bag

Preparation of the patient
Ideally, this procedure should be carried out in conjunction with the daily bed-bath. Give a brief explanation to the patient and ensure privacy.

Procedure
1   Switch off the bedside oscilloscope
2   Detach the electrodes from the oscilloscope patient cable.
3   Gently remove the adhesive tape and the electrodes from the patient.
Ensure the minimum of discomfort to the patient and traction to the electrodes.
4   If non-disposable electrodes are in use, these

should be carefully washed in the warm water to remove the electrode cream and dried using the tissues.

5 Wash (shave if required) and dry the patient's skin area where the electrodes are to be placed. Talcum powder should not be used as this will prevent good adhesive contact with the electrodes.

6 Apply a small amount of the electrode cream to the centre of the electrode and apply to the patient's skin with adhesive tape.

NOTE. The variety of electrodes on the market is numerous. Some are disposable. The manufacturer's instructions should be followed as far as possible.

Position of the electrodes. The electrodes are marked with the initials of the limbs, i.e.

RL—right leg   LL—left leg
RA—right arm   LA—left arm

or by colour coding. The colour coding varies according to the manufacture.

LIMB ELECTRODES. Limb electrodes positioned on the outer aspect of the wrists and the lower leg.

CHEST ELECTRODES. Figure 12 illustrates the sites most commonly used for the positioning of chest electrodes.

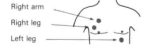

Right arm
Right leg
Left leg

Fig. 12 Positions most commonly used for chest electrodes.

7 Once the electrodes are secured, the cable is connected to the oscilloscope which is then switched on. The size of the complexes on the screen should be approximately 2.5 cm in height. This is adjusted using the sensitivity control.

8 Check the alarm rate limits are set as required before leaving the patient.

Continuing care
The electrodes should be cleaned and replaced once daily or more often if required. Pre-jellied electrodes only require to be replaced every 48 hours unless they become detached.

Careful observation of the patient's skin should be made for any skin irritation made by the electrodes, the adhesive tape or the electrode cream.

Precautions and danger
1 The electrodes must not be removed while the patient is having a dangerous dysrhythmia.

2 Electrode cream with a high sodium content should not be used for continuous monitoring.

3 To prevent injury, limb electrodes should **never** be placed on the inner aspects of the patient's limbs.

4 Defective electrodes must be discarded.

5 **A poor picture on the oscilloscope** may be caused by:

patient movement

too much or too little electrode cream

interference from electrical apparatus, e.g. electric razor

poor electrode contact due to non-shaved area of skin of the male patient

3.52
Examination of the nervous system

3

Examination of the nervous system is carried out to:
    estimate cerebral functions
    test the cranial nerves
    test the motor and sensory nervous systems

Equipment
Patella hammer
Sphygmomanometer
Stethoscope
Pen torch (to test the reaction of pupils to light)
Ophthalmoscope
Auriscope
Tuning forks of varied pitches
Tongue depressor
Small bottles of various substances for taste and smell:

Taste	*Smell*
Sugar	Peppermint
Salt	Perfume
Lemon juice	Coffee
Vinegar	

Cotton wool balls
Small soft brush
Test tubes with hot and cold water
Sterile hypodermic needles (with disposable receptacle)
Asthesiometer (dividers for tactile sensation)
Skin pencil
Tape measure

Familiar objects: coins, thimble, comb (to test for
  recognition, shape, roughness and smoothness)

Preparation of the patient
An explanation is given to the patient. The patient
  should wear light clothing, e.g. pyjamas/night-
  dress, dressing-gown and slippers. No stockings
  or socks should be worn.
The examination is usually carried out in the treatment room.

Procedure
1   The examination is carried out by a doctor. The
nurse may be asked to assist, e.g. with a confused
patient.
2   After the examination the patient is returned to
the ward and made comfortable.

3.53
Central venous pressure

3

A normal central venous pressure exists when the venous system is adequately filled and the cardiac output matches the venous return. **Normal value** is $+5$ to $+10$ cm water.

Readings may be taken at the site of the basilic vein, the external jugular vein and the subclavian vein.

The central venous pressure will be low when the venous return is low after:

haemorrhage

severe burns

severe loss of fluid from the alimentary tract

certain types of septicaemia

The central venous pressure will be high in:

excessive venous returns due to overtransfusion

excessive venous return due to myocardial insufficiency

Equipment

As for Procedure 12.3, Intravenous Therapy plus:

Intravenous catheter 30–45 cm

Venous pressure manometer set including a three-way tap filled with the required fluid, e.g. normal saline 0.9% solution

Centimetre scale taped to the infusion stand

Long ruler with a spirit level attached to its centre

Preparation of the patient

As per Procedure 12.3.

3

Procedure

1   The intravenous catheter is inserted by the doctor into the chosen vein and connected to the previously filled venous pressure manometer set which is taped to the infusion stand with the attached centimetre scale.

2   The three-way tap (see Fig. 13) allows the patient to receive intravenous fluid with the tap in *Position A*. The tap is then turned to *Position B* so that the extension fills about half way up with the fluid from the infusion. The tap is now turned to *Position C* and it will be noted that the level in the extension arm will fall or rise and finally settle at one level.

NOTE. Minor fluctuations in the level should be present with the respiration rate. If these are absent the doctor must be informed, as this means either the catheter is not in the chest or it is blocked.

3   The zero reference line is established as follows:

(a) The level of the manubric-sternal notch is taken and marked.

(b) The metric ruler with the spirit level attached is used to obtain the level of the centimetre scale, i.e. the ruler being placed against the metric scale at one end and the other end resting against the manubric-sternal joint. The spirit level gives the horizontal.

(c) A point 5 cm below this level (the horizontal) represents the *zero reference line*.

4   The central venous pressure is now read as (plus)$+$ or (minus)$-x$ cm of water.

5   Once the central venous pressure has been read, the three-way tap is returned to *Position A* to allow the patient to receive intravenous fluids via the intravenous catheter.

NOTE. The patient may move in bed and the zero

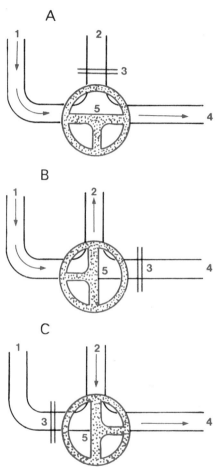

Fig. 13 Three-way tap, showing the positions required to record a patient's central venous pressure: position A enables the patient to receive intravenous fluids; B allows the fluid to pass into the manometer; and C lets the fluid in the manometer pass into the patient and settle at one level. The number keys in all represent: (1) infusion; (2) manometer; (3) closed; (4) patient; (5) three-way stopcock.

reference line should be determined each time before the central venous pressure reading is made.

The frequency and acceptable range of the central venous pressure will be determined by the doctor.

3

Reporting

The doctor must be notified if:

the respiratory fluctuations in the venous manometer are absent (see Note after item 2 of Procedure)

there is a change in the central venous pressure range of indicated acceptable pressures

there is a change in the patient's pulse rate or blood pressure

Special nursing note

The central venous pressure catheter lies in the great veins within the chest. The risk of infection, therefore, is greater than with an ordinary intravenous infusion.

On removal the terminal portion (tip) of the intravenous catheter may be sent to the laboratory for bacteriological examination.

4
Ear, Nose and Throat Nursing Procedures

4

4.1
Ear, nose and throat examination

Equipment
Forehead mirror and standard lamp or head lamp
  or auriscope
Aural speculae ⎱
Nasal sepculae ⎰ of different sizes
Angled aural and nasal forceps
Tuning forks
Tongue depressors
Postnasal mirrors
Spirit lamp and matches (unless disposable mirrors
  are used)
Throat swabs in containers
Tongue holding cloths, e.g. linen or gauze
Wool dressed applicators
Receptacles for soiled instruments
Disposal bag

Preparation of the patient
The procedure is explained to the patient and he/
she should be sitting up, if possible. If necessary the
nurse stands behind the patient and holds his/her
head steady. A small child should sit on his/her
parent's or nurse's knee with the legs and arms held.

Procedure
An ear, nose and throat examination is done by the
doctor who will examine each organ in turn, usually
commencing with either the nose or the throat.

4.2
Proof puncture and antral lavage

4

Proof puncture and antral lavage are routinely carried out in the ear, nose and throat unit. They are normally combined and are used in the diagnosis and treatment of maxillary disease.

Equipment
Source of light
Dental syringe and needle
Cartridge of lignocaine 2% and 1 in 80 000 adrenaline
Nasal speculae of various sizes
Wool dressed applicators
Cotton wool mops
Gauze swabs
Bowl and receiver
Protective covering for the patient
Disposal bag
Trocar and cannulae and Higginson's syringe with an adaptor to fit the cannulae
Jug or bowl of lotion (300 ml at 37.8°C), e.g. normal saline
Lotion thermometer

Preparation of the patient
1   The procedure is explained to the patient.
2   The appropriate part of the patient's nose is anaesthetised by the doctor and the patient is then asked to sit quietly for a short period while the anaesthetic takes effect.
3   The patient is given a bowl in which to spit saliva and also tissue wipes.

Procedure

1   The doctor inserts the trocar and cannula through the inferior meatus into the antrum. He/she then removes the trocar and attaches the Higginson's syringe and adaptor to the cannula.

2   The antrum is gently syringed with the lotion (the temperature of which **must be checked before** administration). The return fluid is collected in a receiver held beneath the patient's nose.

3   On completion of the lavage the doctor removes the cannula or replaces it with polythene tubing if antral drainage or further therapy is required.

4   The patient's nose is wiped and he/she is made comfortable and told that the anaesthetic effects will soon wear off.

5   The returned fluid is examined and a specimen is taken for bacteriological examination if necessary.

6   The specimen is clearly labelled and sent with the appropriate form to the laboratory.

Aftercare of equipment

All used articles are cleaned and washed with detergent and hot water and/or recommended disinfectants, re-sterilised or, if disposable, discarded.

4.3
Anterior nasal packs

Nasal packs may be used to control severe epistaxis.

Equipment
Topical local anaesthetic, e.g. lignocaine 4% and 1 in 1000 adrenaline
Wool dressed applicators
Nasal spray
2.74 m of 1.27 cm or 2.54 cm ribbon gauze
Nasal speculae of various sizes
Nasal angled forceps
Disposal bag
Good light source

Preparation of the patient
The procedure is explained to the patient and reassurance given.

Procedure
1   The patient's nose is anaesthetised.
2   The 2.74 m of ribbon gauze, either dry, vaselined or soaked with bismuth iodiform and paraffin paste, is inserted gently in layers along the floor of the patient's affected nostril until it is completely packed using forceps.
3   The pack is usually left in situ for 24 hours. If it is kept in situ for longer than 24 hours the patient is prescribed prophylactic antibiotics.
    NOTE. Alternative forms of packing to ribbon gauze include:

finger cots packed with ribbon gauze; one of
which is inserted into each nostril

inflatable epistaxis balloons, specially manufac-
tured for this purpose, e.g. Simpson epistaxis
plug

4

4.4
Posterior nasal packs

Posterior nasal packs may also be used to control severe epistaxis.

Equipment
Local anaesthetic
Wool dressed applicators
Nasal speculae of various sizes
Two fine catheters, e.g. size 6 FG
Length of tape about 1.27 cm wide and 60 cm long to the middle of which a small gauze plug is **securely sewn**
Needle, cotton thread and scissors
Tongue depressor
Postnasal mirror (if required)
Nasal angled forceps
Disposal bag
Good light source
Equipment for anterior packing (if required)

Preparation of the patient
The procedure is explained to the patient and reassurance given.

Procedure
1   After the patient's nose has been anaesthetised the catheters are passed through each nostril into the pharynx where they are grasped with forceps and are drawn out through the patient's mouth. Once outside the mouth an end of the tape is securely stitched on to each catheter tip. The catheters

are then drawn back through the patient's mouth, pharynx and nose to the outside where they are removed from the tape ends. The ends of the tape are gently but firmly pulled out of the nose until the gauze plug is felt to lodge in the patient's posterior nares. The ends of the tape are tied neatly and comfortably in front of the patient's nose.

2   An anterior pack will also be inserted, if necessary.

4

4.5
Treatments of the nose

Nasal drops

1   The patient sits or lies with his/her head held back.

2   The drops are checked with the patient's prescription sheet and the prescribed number of drops are instilled into each nostril or nostrils.

3   The patient is asked to keep his/her head extended for a few minutes and is advised not to blow his/her nose for a short time. Excess drops which collect in the patient's throat can be spat out.

4   The patient's medicine recording sheet is completed.

Nasal creams

Nasal creams are applied to the patient's anterior nares with a dressed applicator or from individual small tubes of cream.

Nasal insufflation

As for instillation of nasal drops, only in this instance the medicine is sprayed in powder form into the patient's nose from an insufflator.

Nasal sprays

As for the instillation of nasal drops, only in this instance the nozzle of the medicine container is inserted into the patient's anterior nares and the container is squeezed two or three times to instil the medicine. The procedure is repeated for the patient's other nostril.

4.6
Treatments to the throat

Throat spray
1   The patient's tongue is depressed.
2   The medicine is sprayed on to the lateral and posterior walls of the patient's pharynx from the spray container.

Throat swab
1   In a good light the patient is asked to open his/her mouth as wide as possible.
2   The patient's tongue is depressed and the swab is taken from the area of the tonsils or lateral pharyngeal walls. During this part of the procedure, care must be taken not to touch any part of the mouth or uvula.
3   The swab is then sent in an appropriate labelled container with the correct form to the laboratory.

4.7
Syringing the ear (aural syringing)

Ear syringing is carried out to:

Remove wax. The wax may be softened by instilling Cerumol or warm olive oil or almond oil (36.8°C) a few hours before syringing.

Remove foreign bodies in the external auditory meatus; **only** certain types.

Cleanse the external meatus of discharge in **chronic** otitis media.

Equipment
Good light
Auriscope
Aural syringe
500 ml of warm (36.8°C) lotion, e.g. tap water, normal saline
Lotion thermometer
Warmed receiver for returned fluid
Wool dressed applicators
Angled aural forceps
Wool mops
Protective covering for the patient
Disposal bag

Preparation of the patient
An explanation of the procedure is given to the patient and he/she is asked to sit up. His/her shoulder is covered with the protective covering.

Procedure
1   Inspect the patient's ear with the auriscope and arrange light to shine into the external meatus. Note

the condition of the eardrum (tympanic membrane). If it is perforated **do not syringe**. Report to the nurse in charge.

2 Ask the patient to hold the receiver below his/her ear.

3 Check the temperature of the lotion, fill the aural syringe and expel the air.

4 Straighten the auditory canal by pulling the pinna upwards and backwards (adult).

5 Insert the nozzle of the aural syringe just into the auditory canal, (**do not insert more than 1 cm**) and pointing to the roof or posterior wall of the auditory canal.

6 Inject the fluid gently for discharge or gently with a little force for removal of wax.

7 Repeat item 6 until the return fluid appears clear.

8 Carefully mop the external auditory meatus dry and inspect the patient's ear with the auriscope to see if the wax or discharge has been removed.

9 Remove equipment and leave the patient comfortable.

10 Check return fluid and report the results to the nurse in charge.

Aftercare of equipment
All used articles are cleaned and washed with detergent and hot water and/or recommended disinfectant or if disposable discarded.

4

4.8
Treatments to the ear

4

Medicines instilled or applied to the external auditory meatus are usually in the form of drops or ointments.

Ear drops
1 Mop the meatus and auricle dry with a dressed applicator. **Do not insert** the applicator more than about 1.25 cm into the meatus.
2 Tilt the patient's head sideways to bring the affected ear uppermost.
3 The drops are checked with the patient's prescription sheet and instil sufficient drops (two to three) to fill the meatus. Then press the tragus against the meatal orifice to gently work the drops through the external auditory canal.
4 Ask the patient to remain with his/her head tilted for about 5 minutes, after which the excess drops can be wiped off.
5 A small plug of cotton wool may be inserted, if ordered, just inside the meatus.
6 The patient's medicine recording sheet is completed.

Aural packing
A short strip of ribbon gauze impregnated with a medicine, e.g. 10% ichthyol and glycerine is inserted gently into the meatus with angled aural forceps. This is occasionally used in treating furunculosis.

4.9
Tracheostomy care

A tracheostomy is an operation to create an artificial airway. It may be temporary or permanent. The aperture which remains is the tracheostomy.

Nursing notes

An individual nurse is normally responsible for the management of the patient's nursing care.

The patient is nursed in a position appropriate to his/her condition.

The **equipment** necessary for the care of the tracheostomy is placed on a trolley near the patient's bed.

Writing materials for the patient's use should be on his/her bedside locker.

Equipment

Trolley with:

Tracheal dilators

Two spare tracheostomy tubes (one the same size and one smaller)

Suction catheters of a size not greater than half the diameter of the lumen of the tracheostomy

Suction machine

Sterile disposable gloves

A sterile bowl containing sterile normal saline 0.9% or water

Disposal bag in bin with pedal control

Face masks

Suction
Suction is carried out as often as necessary in the immediate postoperative period.
1   Put on mask and wash and dry hands.
2   Open catheter pack and expose proximal end of the suction catheter and attach to the suction machine tubing and switch on the machine.
3   Wash and dry hands again and put on sterile gloves.
4   Pick up the catheter and by leaving the eyelet uncovered allow its cover to fall free.
    NOTE. Control of the catheter is achieved by the **sterile gloved hand—**the sterility of which **must be maintained—**or by the use of sterile forceps.
5   The catheter is then inserted through the tracheostomy tube down into the bronchial tree for about 10 to 15 cm.
6   The suction is then applied by either occluding the eyelet of the catheter or the open arm of the Y-connection depending on the type of catheter being used.
7   The catheter is gently withdrawn while maintaining suction until it is completely out of the tracheostomy tube.
    NOTE. Contamination of the catheter between insertions **must be avoided**. A fresh catheter is used for each session.
8   The procedure is repeated until most of the secretions have been removed.
9   In some units 5 ml of normal saline 0.9% is inserted into the tracheostomy tube before and after suction. In other units air or oxygen is humidified before entering the trachea.

Tracheostomy tubes
Deflation of the cuff is only carried out if ordered

by the anaesthetist. Care must be taken to ensure that the same amount of air is inserted each time.

Silver tracheostomy tubes. The nurse is responsible for changing the **inner tube** as often as is necessary and replacing it with a clean sterile one. It is advisable to remove the inner tube before carrying out suction. The inner tube is cleaned by passing materials such as ribbon gauze or pipe cleaners through the lumen of the tube after soaking it in bicarbonate of soda or saline solution. The inner tube is then re-sterilised if a duplicate inner tube is available, otherwise it is cleaned thoroughly.

All tubes **must be tied securely** in position by tapes round the patient's neck.

Changing a tracheostomy tube
A plain tracheostomy tube may be changed twice daily. If a disposable cuffed blue line tracheostomy tube is used, this is changed every 1 to 5 days depending on medical staff instructions.

Equipment
Trolley with:
Tracheal dilators
Tracheostomy tube (correct size)
Large dressing pack
2 ml syringe
Normal saline 0.9% (sterile)
Sterile gloves
Sterile towel
Spencer Well's artery forceps (sterile)
Masks
Source of suction

Procedure

As for sterile dressing—see Procedure 3.17 but apply suction before commencing.

1   Assistant unties the tapes from the tracheostomy tube and removes the dressing, deflates the cuff and prepares a new suction catheter.

2   Dresser puts on the sterile gloves and removes the tube using dressing forceps.

3   Assistant applies suction to the stoma.

4   Dresser cleans the stoma with the normal saline 0.9%, inserts the new tracheostomy tube and removes the introducer.

NOTE. If a cuffed tube is used the cuff of the new tracheostomy tube should be inflated several times before it is inserted.

5   Assistant inflates the cuff of the tube while the dresser holds the tube in position. (Use Spence Well's artery forceps while inflating the cuff.)

6   Dresser inserts gauze swabs to either side of the stoma and ties the tube in position.

7   Assistant applies suction using the new catheter.

8   The protective cover is then applied over the tube.

Tracheostomy sutures

Tracheostomy sutures are removed on the seventh day following operation.

Laryngectomy protectors

Laryngectomy bibs are sometimes used when humidification is not required. These are washed in the recommended disinfectant solution and can be used up to nine times.

Care of the stoma while the tracheostomy tube is in situ

Care of the stoma while the tracheostomy tube is in situ is a sterile procedure.

Secretions around the tracheostomy are common in the initial stages following operation and frequent dressing changes are required. These are carefully done by easing the soiled dressing out from around the tube, cleansing the area with swabs or cotton wool buds moistened in normal saline 0.9% and replacing fresh dressing swabs.

NOTE. **Always check** after dressing the stoma that the tapes of the tubes have not become slack. Re-tie using a reef knot.

Care of the stoma after removal of the tracheostomy tube

The stoma is cleaned frequently with normal saline 0.9% and a dry dressing re-applied as necessary.

5
Ophthalmic Nursing Procedures

5

213

5.1
Ophthalmic examination and treatments

Staff carrying out ophthalmic examination and treatment procedures **must have** scrupulously clean hands with short smooth rounded finger nails.

If a patient is blind or has his/her eyes covered it is especially important to carefully explain the steps in the procedure.

Gentle handling of the patient's eyelids is essential.

Always check the patient's chart which will indicate which eye is to be treated.

5

5.2
Eye examination

Equipment

Good light

Ophthalmoscope

Drops to dilate the pupil, if prescribed, e.g. cyclo-
pentolate 0.5 to 1%—instilled prior to eye examination

Drops to constrict the pupil should also be available,
e.g. Pilocarpine 1 to 2%

Preparation of the patient

The procedure is explained to the patient and he/
she is reassured, as necessary.

5.3
Instillation of eye drops

Equipment
Small tray with:
Prescribed eye drops and dropper (these may be
　individual sterile packs)
Ophthalmic swabs
Disposal bag

Preparation of the patient
Explain the procedure to the patient. Have the
patient seated or lying down with his/her head held
backwards.

Procedure
1　Wash and dry hands.
2　Check which eye is to be treated.
3　Gently pull down the patient's lower eyelid with
finger.
4　Ask the patient to look up and instil the prescribed eye drops into the lower fornix, being careful not to touch the patient's eye with the dropper
which should be held about 2.5 cm above the
patient's eye.
5　Gently wipe the area to remove excess moisture
from the inner canthus outwards using a fresh
ophthalmic swab for each stroke.

Aftercare of equipment
1　Clear and clean the tray.
2　Place disposal bag containing used ophthalmic
swabs in appropriate container.

5.4
Instillation of eye creams

Creams are mostly used in the form of single or
multiple dose tubes where a slender ribbon of
cream comes out of the nozzle on applying pressure to the tube.

The nozzle **must not touch** the patient's eye and
the ribbon of cream is drawn from the inner canthus of the patient's eye outwards.

5.5
Bathing or swabbing the eye

Equipment
Tray with:
Eye dressing pack
Sterile lotion, e.g. normal saline 0.9% standing in
a container of water at 37.8°C
Lotion thermometer
Disposal bag

5

Preparation of the patient
Explain the procedure to the patient. Have the
patient seated or lying down in a comfortable position with his/her head held backward.

Procedure
1   Wash and dry hands.
2   Check which eye is to be treated.
3   Check the temperature of the lotion.
4   Open eye dressing pack.
5   Moisten a swab with the lotion using it to gently
swab the patient's eye from inner canthus outwards.
6   Repeat, as often as required, using a clean swab
for each swabbing.
7   Gently dry the area to remove excess moisture.
8   Clear away equipment and ensure the patient is
comfortable.

Aftercare of equipment
As Procedure 5.3.

5.6
Eye irrigation

Eye irrigation is often required to remove corrosives from the eye and, if so, it is an emergency procedure. No time must be lost. Simply cut the top off a Polyfusor normal saline 0.9% container and irrigate the affected eye from the inner canthus outwards. If normal saline is not available tap water can be used. In the case of lime burns the patient's eyelids must be padded.

Equipment
Tray with:
Eye dressing pack
Protection for the patient's shoulders
Bottle of sterile normal saline 0.9% standing in a container of water at 37.8°C
Lotion thermometer
Receiver (kidney shaped) for returned lotion
Irrigator (may be a sterile undine, syringe or Polyfusor bottle)
Disposal bag

Preparation of the patient
Explain the procedure to the patient and place the patient in a comfortable position.
Protect the patient's shoulders.
Ask the patient to hold the receiver against his/her cheek.
Stand behind the patient.

Procedure

1 Test the temperature of the lotion and fill the irrigator.

2 Allow some of the lotion to flow over the patient's cheek to accustom him/her to the temperature of the lotion.

3 Holding the irrigator about 2.5 cm above the affected eye direct the flow over the lower fornix from the inner canthus outwards. Whilst doing this ask the patient to look up, down and all round.

4 Continue until the patient's eye is clean.

5 Gently dry the patient's eyelids and remove the receiver and the protective covering.

6 Clear away equipment and ensure the patient is comfortable.

Aftercare of equipment

As Procedure 5.3.

5

5.7
Socket irrigation

Socket irrigation is similar to eye irrigation (see Procedure 5.6) but the eye prosthesis is removed first. This is done by gently pulling down the lower lid, inserting a small eye spatula under the prosthesis and applying gentle pressure to the upper eyelid.

The eye socket is irrigated with normal saline 0·9%.

The eye prosthesis is washed with chlorhexidine gluconate (Hibitane) 1 in 5000 (0.02%) aqueous solution.

The prosthesis is replaced by gently inserting it towards the inner canthus (the patient may do this) and pressing it gently into place.

5.8
Hot spoon bathing of the eye

Equipment
Tray with:
Large firm based bowl half filled with very hot water
Wooden spoon, padded with cotton wool and covered with tubegauze
Ophthalmic swabs
Disposal bag

Preparation of the patient
Seat the patient comfortably and place the tray on a **firm surface** in front of him/her. Explain the procedure to him reinforcing the importance of safety.

Procedure
1   Check that working surface is firm.
2   Instruct the patient to:
(a) dip the wooden spoon into the bowl of water and to carefully press out excess moisture against the side of the bowl
(b) to lean forward and close his/her eyes and to hold the spoon close but **not touching** the affected eye, until the heat diminishes
(c) re-heat the spoon and continue in this fashion for 5 to 15 minutes
3   Dry the patient's eyelids and cheek.
4   Clear away the equipment and make the patient comfortable.

Aftercare of equipment

1 Clear and clean the tray.
2 Place disposal bag containing used ophthalmic swabs in the appropriate container.
3 Wash and clean the bowl.
4 Wooden spoon is re-padded as required.

6
Gynaecological Nursing Procedures

6

6.1
Vulval toilet

Vulval toilet is the swabbing of the vulva and perineum. It is done: postoperatively in certain gynaecological conditions, for the postpartum patient who is unable to use the bidet and when a bedfast patient is unable to do this herself.

Equipment
Basic trolley for sterile procedures (see Procedure 3.16) plus:
Sterile bowl of lotion, e.g. normal saline, aqueous Savlon 1 in 100 (1% solution)
Vaginal pack
Disposable gloves
Waterproof protection for the bed
Disposal bag

Preparation of the patient
As for urinary catheterisation (see Procedure 3.23) but the patient passes urine before commencement of the procedure. Waterproof protection is placed under the patient's buttocks.

Procedure
1 Take trolley to the bedside and ensure privacy.
2 Wash and dry hands and prepare equipment.
3 The vulva is swabbed from above downwards and from without inwards, using as many swabs as required. The vulva is then dried and a vulval pad folded in half is placed in position, if required.

4 The patient is then turned on her side and the area around the anus is swabbed and dried.

5 The vulval pad is then opened and fixed to a sanitary belt.

6 Allow the patient to wash her hands. Clear away equipment, leave the patient comfortable and un-screen the bed.

Aftercare of equipment
As per Procedure 3.16.

Observations and reporting
Note and report the condition of the area and the presence of any discharge to the nurse in charge.

Nursing note
If perineal sutures are present, the suture line may be swabbed gently using forceps and moist swabs and dried in the same way. The suture line is covered with a sterile pad.

6.2
Vulval douche

A vulval douche consists of pouring warm sterile lotion over the vulva and is carried out for the same purposes as vulval toilet.

Equipment
As for vulval toilet (see Procedure 6.1) plus:
Foil bowl for the lotion, e.g. Savlon 1 in 100 (1% solution) at 37.8°C
Lotion thermometer
Covered bedpan

Preparation of the patient
As per vulval toilet (see Procedure 6.1).

Procedure
As per vulval toilet (see Procedure 6.1) with the exception that the warm lotion is poured from the sterile foil bowl over the vulva into the bedpan. The area is thoroughly dried and a vulval pad applied, if required.

Aftercare of equipment
As per vulval toilet (see Procedure 6.1).

Observations and reporting
As per vulval toilet (see Procedure 6.1).

6.3
Vaginal examination

Equipment
As for vulval toilet (see Procedure 6.1) plus:
Sterile vaginal speculum, e.g. Sim's, Ferguson's, Cusco's (or disposable vaginal speculum) in sterile receiver(s)
Lubrication cream
1 Pair swab holding forceps
Sterile gloves
Angle poise lamp

Preparation of the patient
As for vulval toilet (see Procedure 6.1).
A careful explanation is given to the patient.
The patient's bowel, if possible, should be empty.
Help the patient into one of the following positions:
dorsal with knees apart
left lateral
Sim's
lithotomy

Procedure
1   The vaginal examination is carried out by the doctor.
2   The nurse stays by the patient to afford reassurance and to assist the doctor, when necessary.

Aftercare of equipment
As per Procedure 3.16.

6.4
Vaginal and cervical swabs and smears

Equipment
Disposable gloves—small, medium and large
Disposable speculum
Kidney dish
1 pair sponge holding forceps, e.g. Rampley's
Gauze swabs
Hibitane obstetrical cream in a dispenser
Torch or good source of light
Small disposal bags

6

Cervical smears
The following additional equipment required:
Ayre spatulae
Cytology fixative (glacial acetic acid and ind. meth
  spirit 100%)
Receptacle for fixative
Diamond or lead pencil for marking
Microscope slides
Cytology forms
Blue plastic cytology slide carrier
  NOTE. The smear is taken by the doctor but the
nurse stays with the patient to give reassurance.
  Slides must be left in the cytology fixative for at
least 15 to 20 minutes before placing them in the
special carrier for transportation to the cytology
unit.

High vaginal swabs
The following additional equipment is required:
Sterile throat swab or charcoal swab

Stuart's transport medium
Bacteriology forms
   NOTE. The vulva is swabbed with sterile water,
not antiseptic.

6.5
Vaginal douche

A vaginal douche is the washing out of the vagina
by directing a flow of fluid into the vaginal cavity
and allowing it to flow back by gravity. It is not in
common use but it may be ordered to cleanse the
vagina when there is vaginal discharge or when the
patient is wearing a supportive pessary.

Equipment
Basic trolley for sterile procedures (Procedure 3.16)
 plus:
Vaginal pack
Lotions at 37.8°C, e.g. aqueous Hibitane in 1000
 (0.1%); Cetavlon in 100 (1%); Betadine 1 in 10
 (10%); for radiation vaginitis use Predsol Lotion
 thermometer (chemically disinfected)
Disposable vaginal douche pack
1.7 litre polythene bag with attached clear tubing
Nozzle
Waterproof protection for the bed
Covered bedpan
Disposal bag
Portable intravenous fluid stand

Preparation of the patient
The procedure is carefully explained to the patient
and her cooperation obtained. The patient is offered
a bedpan to pass urine and then she is assisted into
the dorsal position.

Procedure
1 Take the trolley to the bedside and ensure
privacy.

233

2 The bed is protected with the waterproof protection and the warmed bedpan is placed in position.
3 Nurse(s) wash and dry hands.
4 **Assistant** opens packs, tests temperature of lotion and pours it out into appropriate container.
5 Apparatus is connected.
6 The patient's vulva is swabbed as per vulval toilet (see Procedure 6.1).
7 The labia minora are separated and the douche nozzle is gently inserted **downwards and backwards** over the posterior vaginal wall for about 7 to 8 cm.
8 The lotion is allowed to run in and the nozzle is rotated gently during the procedure to allow the fluid to reach all the fornices.
9 When the return fluid is clear the nozzle is removed and the apparatus is placed in a disposal bag. The patient is helped to sit up and asked to cough to help drain out any lotion still in the vagina.
10 The patient's vulva is swabbed dry.
11 The bedpan is removed and covered.
12 The patient is assisted on to her side and the perineum is swabbed dry. A vulval pad is fixed into position, if required.
13 Clear away equipment, leave the patient comfortable and unscreen the bed.

Aftercare of equipment
As per Procedure 3.16.

Observations and reporting
Note and report character of the return fluid, condition of the area and the presence of any discharge to the nurse in charge.

6.6
Medicated vaginal pessaries

Vaginal pessaries are cones or balls of cocoa butter or paraffin, or tablets of lactose impregnated with a medicine. They vary in size and shape. Some are supplied with introducers.

Types
Local astringent, e.g. tannic acid
Antiseptic, e.g. penotrane
Antifungal, e.g. nystatin
Antibiotic, e.g. penicillin
Hormonal, e.g. stilboestrol
Local anaesthetic, e.g. locan

6

Equipment
As for vulval toilet (see Procedure 6.1) if required, plus:
Disposable gloves or finger cots
Disposal bag
Prescribed pessary, checked as per medicine prescription sheet

Preparation of the patient
As per vulval toilet (see Procedure 6.1).

Procedure
1 Take equipment to the bedside and ensure privacy.
2 Wash and dry hands.
3 The patient's vulva is swabbed if necessary.
4 The pessary is held in the protected fingers or

introducer and inserted into the patient's vagina as far as comfortably possible.

5   Apply a perineal pad is required.

6   Ask the patient to lie fairly flat in bed for an hour or so to assist in retention of the pessary.

7   Clear away equipment, leave the patient comfortable and unscreen the bed.

Aftercare of the patient

As per Procedure 6.1 if vulva swabbed. If not, disposal bag placed in the appropriate container.

Observations and reporting

1   Complete medicine recording sheet.

2   Note condition of the vulva and the presence of any discharge and report to the nurse in charge.

3   Note later if the pessary has been retained and report to the nurse in charge.

6.7
Supportive vaginal pessaries

Supportive vaginal pessaries are made of vulcanite, rubber or plastic in various shapes and are inserted into the vagina to correct and maintain the position of the uterus. A ring pessary or rubber watch spring pessary is used for correction of uterine prolapse. A Hodge pessary is used for correction of uterine retroversion.

Equipment
As for vulval toilet (see Procedure 6.1) plus:
Sterile pessary
Sterile gloves
Lubricant jelly

Preparation of the patient
As per vulval toilet (see Procedure 6.1).

Procedure
1   Pessary is inserted by a doctor.
2   The patient is dried well.
3   The nurse stays with the patient to afford reassurance.

Aftercare of equipment
As per vulval toilet (see Procedure 6.1).
   NOTE. Insertion of the pessary must be recorded in the patient's Kardex.
The pessary will be changed when necessary, e.g. 12 weeks.

7
Orthopaedic Nursing Procedures

7

7.1
Splints

Splints are used:
  to immobilize various parts of the body in a
    desired position
  to help maintain traction
  as a means of support
  to correct or prevent deformity
Examples of splints in common use are:
  plaster of Paris
  Thomas' bed splint—full or half ring
  metal cock-up splint
  inflatable splint
  plastazote

General nursing points
When used to immobilise fractures, the joints above
  and below the injury should be immobilised.
Guard against undue pressure on bony promi-
  nences.
Observe for signs that the splint may be too tight.

7.2
Application of a plaster of Paris

Plaster of Paris is the most commonly used form of splintage.

Equipment

Plaster of Paris bandages and slabs (various widths)
Bucket of tepid water (30°C)
Stockinette or tube grip
Wool bandage, e.g. Velband
Orthopaedic felt (plain)
Cling bandage, e.g. Crinx
Skin pencil
Plaster knife
Plaster scissors
Disposable polythene sheeting for protection of the
    patient and the plaster trolley
Protective aprons for the staff
Rubber boots or overshoes for the staff
*If the patient is to stay in bed the following additional
equipment is required:*
    bowl of water
    soap in a dish
    cloth and a towel
    protected pillow
    bed cradle (cage)

Preparation of the patient

The procedure is explained to the patient and his/
her personal clothing protected or covered, as
necessary. The patient is placed in a comfortable
position with the part to which the plaster is to be
applied well supported by the assistant (nurse or
other).

Procedure

1 The skin of the affected area is protected by a length of ribbed stockinette longer than the plaster or a single layer of 'Velband'. Extra padding is required over bony prominences.

2 The first few centimetres of the appropriate plaster bandage is loosened and the bandage is immersed in the bucket of tepid water until the air bubbles cease. The bandage is then removed and gently squeezed to remove excess water and plaster before it is applied.

OR

The plaster bandages are cut to size and shape of a slab which is then gathered in two hands and immersed in the bucket of tepid water until the air bubbles cease. The slab is then removed and gently squeezed to remove excess water and plaster before it is applied.

3 The plaster (bandage or slab) is applied smoothly and gently avoiding dents, tight bands and creases. The edges of the plaster are trimmed and smoothed.

4 The patient's skin around the plaster is washed, rinsed and carefully dried.

5 Instructions are given to the patient on the care and drying of the plaster.

Aftercare of the patient

1 The affected limb is rested on a firm protected pillow and the mattress supported by fracture boards, when necessary. A bed cradle is required in the instance of application of plaster of Paris to the lower limbs.

2 Immediately after the plaster is applied and before it is dry, care **must be taken** not to allow any movements of the joints when transporting or moving the patient into bed as the plaster may crack.

3 When plaster of Paris is applied to the lower limb a protected pillow is placed lengthwise under the lower limb to elevate the heel for the patient's comfort and to aid drying of the plaster.

4 In the instance of spinal plasters the natural curve of the spine is supported with protected pillows until the plaster is dry.

5 Allow free circulation of air around the plaster to assist its drying.

6 Instruct the patient to exercise the exposed digits (fingers, toes) at frequent intervals, e.g. hourly.

Report immediately any signs of cyanosis, oedema, changes in sensation, pain or loss of movement to the nurse in charge.

If the patient complains of pain or burning sensation **under** the plaster report at once to the nurse in charge.

NOTE. If necessary, a plaster can be split, but this should **never** be undertaken on the nurse's own initiative.

7 **Before discharge** ensure that the patient understands that the plaster should not be wet, cut, heated or otherwise interferred with. The patient **must report back at once** if the plaster cracks, becomes loose or uncomfortable; if he/she experiences any pain or discharge occurs; or if fingers or toes become numb, difficult to move, swollen and discoloured.

7.3
Plaster of Paris—definitions and special notes

Bi-valve plaster: to bi-valve a plaster is to cut along its length both laterally and medially.

Window a plaster: to window a plaster a part of it is removed to allow access to an injured area (e.g. suture removal) or to relieve suspected pressure. The window **must be replaced** tightly.

Padded plaster: is where plasterwool or some similar material is placed around the limb prior to the application of the plaster of paris.

Skin-tight plaster: is where stockinette is applied to the limb prior to the application of the plaster of Paris. **Such a plaster can only be used when all swelling has disappeared** (the patient is usually ready to walk at this stage). Certain skin-tight plasters may be applied without stockinette.

Special notes

It is important to have a plaster **smooth inside** rather than highly polished and smooth outside.

Weight should not be put on a lower limb unless it is a walking plaster, i.e. a plaster fitted with a suitable walking base. A walking plaster should not be used for 48 hours by which time it will be thoroughly dry.

7.4
Removal of a plaster of Paris

Equipment
Plaster scissors
Plaster shears
Plaster benders
Plaster saw
Plaster knife
Skin pencil
Disposable polythene sheeting

Preparation of the patient
The procedure is explained to the patient, his/her personal clothing protected and covered, as necessary and he/she is placed in a comfortable position.

Procedure
1   The area of cutting is marked.
2   The plaster is carefully cut using the appropriate instruments and the plaster is removed. The **cutting must not be** hurried and **care must be** taken not to cut the patient's skin.
3   The skin of the former plaster area is washed, rinsed and dried.

7.5
Traction

Traction is a pull exerted on a part of a limb against a pull or thrust of comparable strength in the opposite direction.

Fixed traction is traction exerted on the part of a limb lying between *two fixed points*, e.g. the end of the splint and the ischial tuberosity.

Balanced traction is traction exerted on the part of a limb lying between *two mobile points* which are separated by a pulley or a raised block, e.g. the weights attached to the ends of the splint and the patient's body weight.

Types of traction
Skeletal traction a pin is passed through the bone and the pull (traction) is applied directly to the bone.

Skin traction the pull (traction) is applied to the skin and is transmitted through the soft tissues to the bone.

7.6
Application of skeletal traction

Procedure
The procedure is carried out in theatre conditions and a pin is inserted through the bone. The most common site used is the upper end of the tibia to secure traction on the femur. A local or general anaesthetic is administered.

Procedure after insertion
The sharp end of the pin is protected. A 'U' loop and a stirrup are attached to the projecting ends of the pin. The cord attached to the 'U' loop passes to the pulley and weight at the elevated bed end, this gives *traction*. The cord attached to the stirrup passes to an overhead beam and so to the bed end where the attached weights provide *suspension*.

Nursing observations
The pin. Report any signs of inflammation, discharge or movement of the pin to the nurse in charge.

Traction. Cords and pulleys **must be free** and smooth running. Cords should not be frayed or knotted. Weights should be secure and hanging freely.

Inspection. Check the patient's foot and leg for swelling, blueness, loss of power. Ensure that stirrup and the 'U' loop are not pressing on the patient's skin.

7.7
Application of skin traction

Skin traction is often used in conjunction with a *Thomas' splint*.

Equipment
Bed and fracture boards
Bed elevator
Balkan beam and fittings
Splints of the correct size (if necessary)
Weights and carriers
Tape measure
Skin traction kit (consisting of orthopaedic strapping, spreader and extension cord)
Strong blunt pointed scissors
Cotton wool bandages on tube grip
Adhesive and plain orthopaedic felt
Domette bandages 10 or 15 cm
Adhesive strapping 2.5 cm
Requirements for shaving the limb (if required)
Tincture of benzoin spray
Elastocrepe bandages 10 or 15 cm
Bowl of warm water (33–35°C)
Cloth and towel

Preparation of the patient
The procedure is explained to the patient and reassurance given.

Procedure
1   The patient's limb is gently washed, dried (shaved as required) then sprayed with tincture of benzoin.

2   The orthopaedic strapping is applied down the lateral aspects of the patient's limb ensuring that no creases are present. Any bony prominences are protected by orthopaedic felt or padding.

3   The extension strapping is applied along the length of the leg, cutting it where necessary to fit the circumference of the patient's limb.

4   The spreader should not be less than 5 cm from the patient's foot (in which position the foam lining protects the ankle and side of the patient's foot from pressure).

NOTE. Instructions for the use of skin traction parts should be read before commencing the application of the extension.

5   An elastocrepe bandage is applied over the strapping and fixed with adhesive tape.

NOTE. Pins or clips should not be used for fixing a circular bandage on a limb.

6   The cord is passed over the pulley and attached to the weights if *sliding traction* or tied to a splint if *fixed traction*.

NOTE. Skin extension may be used in conjunction with a Thomas' splint (see Procedure 7.9, Thomas' bed splint).

7.8
Ventfoam extension

Equipment

As per Procedure 7.7 with the exception of the skin traction kit but with the addition of:

Plain felt 7.5 cm

Ventfoam bandage

Special ventfoam spreader

Elastocrepe bandage 15 cm

These additional articles are usually supplied in a special kit.

Procedure

The application is similar in principle as for elastoplast skin extension (Procedure 7.7, Application of skin traction). This may be used when the patient is sensitive to elastoplast.

7

7.9
Thomas' bed splint

Measuring for correct size of splint

1   Measure obliquely round the top of the patient's thigh. An accurate fit is important.

2   Measure from the adductor tendon in the patient's groin to the lowest point on the medial border of the heel.

3   Add 15–20 cm in length for a child. Add 25–30 cm in length for an adult.

4   State whether the splint is for the left or right leg.

NOTE. Certain spints are designed to be used on either leg.

Care of the splint when in use

The ring is washed daily with soap and water, rinsed and dried and dusted with talcum powder or as per manufacturer's instructions. If well enough the patient may be able to do this.

The patient's skin under the ring should be kept dry and moved regularly to prevent pressure sores. The patient can be taught to do this.

Care of the splint when not in use

The ring is washed with leather soap and a protective ointment is applied before storage. **No** spirit, lotions or creams should be used which could make the ring covering brittle, and thus become a potential cause of pressure sores.

Where modern synthetic materials are used instead of leather, these should be washed and dried before storage or as per manufacturer's instructions.

7.10
Nursing management and care related to skin traction and Thomas' splint

Thomas' splint
When a Thomas' splint is used the weight of the patient's limb is borne by slings made of calico. The free end of the splint is supported either by a crucifix or Balkan beam.

Pressure
Pressure may occur at the ankle and the knee of the affected leg due to bandages and extensions. It may occur at the knee or heel of the patient's other leg due to friction. The skin under the ring of a Thomas' splint should be moved every hour (see Procedure 7.9).

A bed cradle is used to support the weight of the bed clothes.

Traction and extensions
The cords and pulleys should run freely. Weights should be hanging free. Bed elevation must be continuous. Bandages should be secure and un-wrinkled—they should be checked regularly to ensure they are not exerting uneven pressure on the patient's leg. The heel of the affected leg should hang free over the sling.

Inspection of the foot
Colour: note for discoloration or excessive whiteness and report
Temperature: compare it with the other foot

Sensation: report complaint of numbness, tingling or pain

Swelling: may indicate too tight bandaging

Power: test full range of ankle movements against resistance, compare with movements of the patient's other foot and report

Restlessness

If the patient is restless during the night suspect a sore or inefficient immobilisation. Check the body temperature, any complaint of pain, burning or changes in sensation and report.

Complaints

Always investigate and report patient complaints. Pain or discomfort could indicate pressure on a nerve. Itching may mean that the patient is developing a reaction to the extension.

Nursing in bed

As patients are often nursed in the head down position due to elevation of the foot of the bed, some may have difficulty in eating and micturating. Assistance should be given in feeding where necessary and a high fluid intake is conducive to a satisfactory urinary bladder function.

Difficulties are also encountered in the use of bedpans. These must be carefully placed in position and the patient must be adequately cleaned after use of a bedpan.

Initially patients may have difficulty in sleeping in the head down position.

Removal of extensions

The elastoplast extension is removed by damping and by easing off gently. Rippling the elastoplast off too quickly may lead to removal of the underlying skin.

8
Paediatric Nursing Procedures

8

Children are different

Care for the total needs of the child may be as important as the care for the immediate problem. If an adult goes into hospital the separation from home, changes in routine, boredom, food etc. may be of secondary importance. For a child, living completely in the present, unable to conceive of the day after tomorrow, the position is quite different.*
Special understanding of the child, parents and the whole family background is therefore essential.

The psychological preparation for procedures and their particular handling is of increased importance, as is meticulous attention to detail, the prevention of mishap and the general surroundings in which the child is treated.

The fact that most procedures may be attended or assisted by the child's mother or father may be alien to the non-paediatric nurse but it is a fact that parents can greatly help in the practical situation and the experienced nurse will soon decide which parents will help and which (a small minority) would be better not to attempt to.

It should be remembered that when children come into hospital they do not suddenly become the property of the nursing staff—they still belong to their parents. Nursing and medical staffs are here to help the parents get the child better. Once this is understood it becomes easy to include parents in every aspect of the child's care and treatment and to gain their cooperation and confidence in us. Thus

* From the Report on the Committee on Child Health Services *Fit for the Future.*

shared care between parents and hospital staff is achieved to the greater satisfaction of all.

Children require as much explanation as possible. This should be **simple, honest** and **reassuring** always pointing towards making him/her better so that he /she can go home. Often it is possible to go through the procedure with teddy or a doll. In reverse the child may act out his/her own fears, frustration etc. through teddy or dolly and nurses should be particularly observant for and attentive to these conversations which can be very revealing.

The play area in a children's ward should always have a hospital corner where items such as stethoscopes, auroscope, syringes (without needles), patella hammer, drip-set, medicine measure etc. can be freely handled and used on dolls or on each other. This will do much to allay fears of the treatment room.

The checking and administration of medicines is of **paramount importance.** Marginal errors in administration to an adult may have little consequence but to a child such errors may prove fatal. This is particularly the case in the administration of intravenous fluid, where overloading of the circulatory system of a small child may happen so quickly and so easily with such disastrous results.

This short introduction to the paediatric nursing section is simply an outline of the more subtle differences between the care of the adult and that of the child. Much more can be found in textbooks and will be learned in practice. Suffice to say that, having read it, the nurse will recognise that:

Children are vulnerable and can be at risk.

Children are unpredictable and require detailed observation.

Children are individuals who require special care.
Children come from families who require under-
standing and support.
Children are a challenge and very rewarding to
nurse.
BUT
Children are different.

8.1
Baby bathing

Equipment

Clean clothes, nappies, cot or bed linen, towels and
   barrier gown
Baby's individual tray with:
Thermometer and Steritemp sleeves
Tube of soft white paraffin (for lubrication of ther-
   mometer if rectal temperature)
Cotton wool balls and buds
Talcum powder
Barrier cream or suitable application for the but-
   tocks
'Infracare' soap, as applicable
Hair brush
Disposal bag and paper towel
Baby bath
Bath thermometer
Scales

Procedure

1   Close all nearby windows and doors to ensure
there are no draughts.
2   Collect all equipment and arrange around the
bath.
3   Wash hands, put on gown and wash hands again.
4   Line the weighing basket with a paper towel or
suitable protection.
5   Gently and carefully undress the baby. If bathing coincides with taking and recording temperature, pulse and respiration (TPR) this should be
done at this point in the procedure.
6   Weigh the baby naked using same machine

each time and get the weight checked if required, record on the appropriate chart.

7   Carefully wrap the baby in a towel and place in a pram or a suitable place while the cot or bed is made with clean linen.

8   Fill the bath and add 'Infracare' (one squeeze). Test the temperature of the water (37°C).

9   Hold the baby under your left arm gently supporting his/her head in your left hand. Gently swab the baby's eyes using the cotton wool balls, using each cotton wool ball **once** only swabbing from the inner canthus outward. Discard each cotton wool ball as used.

10   Wash the baby's face, ears and hair and dry gently. Clean baby's nostrils.

11   Sit comfortably at the bath and immerse the baby in the water with your left hand under the baby's shoulder holding gently the baby's left arm and your right hand under the baby's legs holding the left leg. When the baby is immersed in the water release your **right hand only.**

12   Bath the baby in a systematic manner and after bathing is complete slip your right hand under the baby's legs holding the legs and lift him/her out of the bath onto your towel-covered lap.

13   Dry the baby using a patting movement paying particular attention to skin folds and lightly apply talcum powder to same.

14   Apply cream to the buttock area, if required and put on a clean nappy.

15   Dress the baby in clean clothes.

16   Gently brush the baby's hair.

17   Place the baby back in the clean cot/bed with suitable toys or mobile (see Procedure 1.2, paediatric nursing notes).

18   Clear away equipment.

Aftercare of equipment

Place used clothes, nappy, towels and cot/bed linen in appropriate containers.

Place disposal bag in appropriate container.

Clean and wash all non-disposable equipment including the tray with detergent and hot water and/or recommended disinfectant.

Reset the baby's individual tray.

Observation and reporting

Record and report any abnormalities on baby's skin or behaviour.

Record on the feed chart whether or not the baby had passed urine or had a bowel movement.

NOTE. Remember when handling babies and small children they derive pleasure from being spoken to. They will respond (unless too ill) even if they cannot answer directly and the eye to eye contact plus recognition of their own nurses' voices will not only stimulate them but provide in some measure for them a sense of security which is lacking if mother or father is not present.

8.2
Routine baby care

Equipment
Contents at cot:
Disposable bowl
Disposable gallipot
Soft paper tissues
Cotton wool balls
Sterzac powder in a foil tray
Mediswabs in a foil tray
Barrier gown
At hand on trolley:
   Sterifield sheets
   clean baby linen
   extra cotton wool balls
   thermometer (low reading)
   Steritemp sleeves
   tube of soft white paraffin
   disposal paper bags
   large paper bag on stand for soiled disposable
     goods
   baby linen bag for soiled linen

Procedure
The infant's mother should be shown how to carry
out routine baby care where possible.
1 Close all nearby windows and doors to ensure
that there are no draughts.
2 Collect gallipot and warm water in bowl and set
them on the working area. Place clean linen, Sterifield sheet and disposal bag on second step of cot.
3 Wash hands, put on barrier gown and wash
hands again.

4   Gently and carefully undress the baby and lay on Sterifield sheet. Check baby's identity label.

5   With damp cotton wool ball swab the infant's face and gently dry with dry cotton wool ball.

6   **Check** mouth and behind ears, under chin, neck and under arms. Clean cord with Mediswab and apply Sterzac powder.

7   Take and record rectal temperature.

8   Clean buttocks with damp cotton wool ball and dry with cotton wool ball. Apply cream, if required. Put on a clean nappy.

9   Dress the baby in clean clothes.

NOTE. Enquiries are made at this time of the mother about the baby's feeding and state of stools. Feeding chart is checked and kept up to date.

10   Clear away equipment.

Aftercare of equipment
As per Procedure 8.1.

Nursing notes
Demonstration bath on third post-delivery day. Mothers are encouraged to bath infants under supervision from the fourth post-delivery day onwards (soap to be used).

8.3
Taking and recording temperature

Babies under one year
Preparation
1   Wash hands, put on gown, rewash hands.
2   Unfasten the baby's nappy and change if wet or soiled.
3   Place the thermometer in the Steritemp sleeve and lubricate the tip with soft white paraffin.

Procedure
1   Holding the baby's legs flexed against his/her abdomen with your left hand insert the tip of the thermometer into the baby's anus 1–2.5 cm.
2   Hold the thermometer in position for 3 full minutes.
3   Remove the thermometer, read and record.

Aftercare
1   Clean off excess paraffin from the baby's anus, replace nappy and leave him/her comfortable.
2   Remove the Steritemp sleeve, shake down the thermometer and return the thermometer to the baby's individual tray.
3   Take off gown and wash hands.
   NOTE. All children having rectal temperatures taken must have their own thermometers. These are kept with the baby's toilet requisites in the locker.

Children over one year
Preparation
1   Wash hands.

2 Place the thermometer in the Steritemp sleeve.
3 Unfasten the child's clothes.

Procedure
1 Place the thermometer under the child's axilla. Sit a small toddler on your knee and hold the arm in position.
2 Keep the thermometer in position for 3 full minutes while talking to the child.
3 Remove the thermometer, read and record.

Aftercare
1 Re-fasten the child's clothes and allow him/her to play.
2 Remove the Steritemp sleeve, shake down the thermometer and replace it in the receptacle in the designated storage area, e.g. clean utility room.

NOTE. Body temperature is **never taken orally** in a child as he/she may bite through the glass.

Thermometer **must never be left** within the reach of small children, e.g. locker tops.

It should also be remembered that the thermometers are a carrier source of infection, therefore careful handling is essential.

8.4
Taking and recording the pulse and respirations

The pulse
Sites where the pulse may be taken in a child are:
   radial
   temporal
   apex beat
1   Settle the child and explain the procedure.
2   Count the pulse for a full minute.
3   Record on the appropriate chart and report any differences to the nurse in charge.

Respiration in babies
1   Expose the baby's chest and abdomen by loosening clothing.
2   The movement of the baby's chest and abdomen should be observed.
3   Count for 1 full minute.
4   Record respiration rate on the appropriate chart.
5   Replace the baby's clothing.

Respiration in children
1   Expose the child's chest by loosening clothing.
2   Count respiration for a full minute.
3   Record respiration rate on the appropriate chart.
4   Replace the child's clothes.
   NOTE. It is often easier and wiser to count the pulse and respiration rates of infants and small children before disturbing them if they are resting.
   Do not count the pulse or respirations while the child is crying.

8.5
Urine collection in children

Types
Bag urine
Catheter specimen of urine
Dip slide collection of urine
Midstream specimen of urine
Suprapubic stab urine collection
NOTE. **All** procedures must be explained to the child and reassurance given.

Where possible these procedures should be carried out in the treatment room.

Bag urine
A bag of urine is collected from babies and small children who are not potty trained.
1 It is preferable to apply the urine collection bag over the genital area after the child is bathed. If the procedure is done at another time the child's genital area must be swabbed with warm water (37°C) and thoroughly dried with sterile swabs.
2 The urine collection bag is applied ensuring that it has adhered to the child's skin.
3 The child should be watched carefully and its nappy left off until the specimen of urine has been obtained.
4 Mitts may help to prevent the urine collection bag from being removed.

Catheter specimen of urine
A catheter specimen of urine is carried out as in adults (see Procedure 3.25) but the apprehensive

child may require to be prescribed sedation. Every child will need reassurance and a simple but thorough explanation of what is to happen.

The size of the catheter will depend on the size of the child—these are usually from size 8 FG to 12–14 FG.

Instruments are never used for catheterisation but the nurses should wear sterile gloves. Two or three nurses may be required during catheterisation as the child will need constant support and perhaps to be held firmly.

Dip slide collection of urine

1   A dip slide collection of urine is done as for midstream specimen of urine (see Procedure 3.22) until the urine is collected in the sterile bowl.

2   Then remove the cap from the dip slide bottle and dip the attached slide into the freshly collected urine ensuring that the slide is completely immersed.

3   Return the slide to the bottle without touching the slide surface and secure the cap of the bottle tightly.

NOTE. The surface of the dip slide should be 'slimy' before it is used. If it is dry the specimen may be of no use.

Do not refrigerate dip slide specimens.

Midstream specimen of urine

Obtained as per adults (see Procedure 3.22)

Suprapubic stab urine collection

A suprapubic stab urine collection is done by a doctor and is used when there is difficulty in obtaining a clean bag urine.

Equipment
Basic trolley for sterile procedures (Procedure 3.16) plus:
    5 ml syringe and a No. 21 G needle
    Universal container (for urine)
    Sterile gloves
    Hand towel

Procedure
1   Prior to the procedure sedation may be prescribed for the child.
2   The procedure is carried out by the doctor assisted by the nurse.
3   The child is held firmly.
4   The skin over the child's suprapubic area is cleansed thoroughly.
5   The doctor inserts the needle into the urinary bladder and aspirates urine
6   The needle is withdrawn and a small dressing applied.
7   The specimen of urine is placed in the universal container and sent to the laboratory.
8   The child is made comfortable and the equipment is removed.

Aftercare of equipment
As per Procedure 3.16.

8.6
Rectal lavage

Rectal lavage is the washing out of the rectum in preparation for examination such as barium studies, proctoscopy and sigmoidoscopy and prior to rectal surgery.

NOTE. An **evacuant enema** may be necessary prior to the lavage to clear the rectum of solid matter, but should **never be given** in suspected cases of Hirschprung's disease to infants under the age of 12 months.

Equipment
Trolley with:

Top shelf:
Measuring jug containing normal saline 0.9% solution at 37°C (can be made by mixing one level 5 ml spoon of salt (sodium chloride) in 540 ml of water)
Lotion thermometer
Funnel, tubing (approximately 45 cm in length) and straight connection already assembled
Rubber or disposable rectal catheter—size suitable to the patient 5-24 FG (18-14 EG)
Lubricant
Medical wipes
Receptacle for soiled apparatus
Disposal bag

Bottom shelf:
Bucket for returned fluid
Additional saline solution

Waterproof protection for the bed and the floor
Polythene apron and barrier gown for the nurse

Preparation of the child
Careful and adequate preparation of the child is of
    the utmost importance as the rectal lavage may be
    prolonged and require repeating daily until the
    child's bowel is adequately cleansed.
Sedation may be prescribed for small or apprehen-
    sive children.
Toys or books should be brought with the child.
Transistor radio is often helpful.

Procedure
1   Requires two nurses. Take the trolley to the
bedside or bathroom and ensure privacy.
2   Turn back the top bed clothes and place the
child in the left lateral position, with gown rolled
well up or pyjama trousers removed. Keep the child
warm by placing a blanket over the shoulders and
back and another blanket over the legs.
3   Protect the bed by placing waterproof sheeting
under the child's buttocks.
4   Place waterproof protection on the floor and
stand the bucket on it.
5   Lubricate the terminal 5–10 cm of the catheter
and gently insert through the anal sphincter into the
rectum for 5–10 cm to release any flatus.
6   Test the temperature of the normal saline 0.9%
solution. This should be 37°C.
7   Run through a small amount of the solution to
expel the air in the assembled apparatus. Kink the
tubing and connect to catheter in situ.
8   The fluid in the funnel of the assembled apparatus is allowed to run slowly into the child's rectum.
    NOTE. The amount of fluid used in each cycle
depends on the age and size of the child. As little as

60 ml may be used in small children and infants increasing to 300 ml in, e.g. a 10 year old child.

9   When the funnel is almost empty lower it to the floor level in an upright position until the full amount of the fluid has been syphoned (returned). Kink the tubing and invert the funnel to empty contents into the bucket.

10   Refill the funnel with a further supply of the saline solution before raising it 30 cm or so above the level of the mattress.

NOTE. Repeat the cycle (items 8–10) until the fluid returned is clear.

11   Then gently withdraw the catheter through a medical wipe placed over the child's anus while holding the funnel at a lower level. (This allows any retained fluid to be syphoned.)

12   Place the apparatus in the receptacle on the trolley.

13   The child is left clean, dry and comfortable. (If the procedure has been long it is often more comforting to give the child a warm bath.)

NOTE. The child should be praised for being co-operative and reassurance provided, if required.

14   Unscreen the bed and remove equipment.

Aftercare of equipment
Place disposal bag and contents into appropriate container. Thoroughly wash and clean all non-disposable equipment with detergent and hot water and/or recommended disinfectant.

NOTE. The contents of the bucket are examined, measured and disposed of and the result recorded in the child's nursing Kardex.

Wash hands thoroughly.

8.7
Colonic lavage

Colonic lavage is the washing out of the colon and is used prior to colonic surgery and in Hirschsprung's disease.

Procedures

The procedure ordered by the doctor is essentially the same as for rectal lavage (see Procedure 8.6) with the following exceptions:

1   Larger volumes of normal saline 0.9% are necessary.

2   The rectal catheter is inserted for a greater distance than that used in the rectal lavage procedure, i.e. 20–30 cm.

3   Irrigation and syphonage is performed with the child in the right and left lateral positions and may be required in the supine position as well.

NOTE. The importance of using normal saline (isotonic solution) for the procedures of rectal lavage and colonic lavage in children is paramount, since the use of large quantities of water, which might well be absorbed (particularly in Hirschsprung's disease) can lead to water intoxication, cerebral oedema with fits and subsequent brain damage.

Children having intensive colonic lavage daily may develop sudden, otherwise unexplained, rises in body temperature. This is the so called washout reaction and must be reported immediately and the washouts discontinued *pro tem*. Other symptoms which may arise and for which the nurse must be alert are vomiting, headache and increased weight gain—for this reason such children should be carefully weighed each day.

8

8.8
Wound dressing using Hampshire dressing

See also Procedures 3.17 and 3.18.

Equipment
Trolley prepared as per Procedure 3.16
Hampshire dressing packet
Small dressing pack
Scissor set
Skin cleansing lotion
Material to secure dressing/s, e.g. zinc oxide strapping, bandages, elastoplast
Micropore
Hand towel
Mask/s
Additional items as required for specific procedures

Preparation of the child
Wound dressing should be carried out, where possible, in the treatment room, away from other children.

The child **must be told** what is to happen and reassured.

If parents want to stay with their child during the procedure they must wear clean gowns and masks and understand the procedure fully.

Procedure
1 Loosen material used to secure the dressing.
2 Put on mask. Wash and dry hands and open the

Hampshire pack by grasping the loose flaps and peeling apart to the bottom seal.

3   Lay the pack on the clean surface of the trolley so that the contents fall onto the inner surface of the printed flap. Alternatively the contents of the pack can be dropped onto a sterile surface on the trolley.

4   Grasp the loose edge of the plastic bag from the pack and insert right hand. Punch thumb into one of the bottom corners of the bag and fingers into the other corner.

5   Pick up the soiled dressing and invert the plastic bag to enclose the soiled dressing. Remove the paper covering from the adhesive tape on the bag flap and attach the bag to the edge of the trolley.

6   Wash hands and forearms thoroughly, dry thoroughly using the hand towel. Put on sterile gloves and carry out the dressing procedure.

7   Arrange sterile equipment in order of use on the upper shelf of the trolley. Remove forceps from the small dressing pack and lay them aside as they will not be used.

8   **Using gloved hands instead of forceps** drape the wound area and swab the wound area as for basic dressing procedure (see Procedure 3.17) and proceed in this manner with the dressing as instructed.

9   When the dressing is completed remove the gloves and place them in the plastic bag. Clear away equipment.

10   The child is returned to the ward or play area and suitably rewarded, as necessary.

Aftercare of equipment
See Procedure 3.16.

   NOTES. **Do not allow** gloved hands to touch the patient's skin while carrying out the procedure.

Use gloved right hand for cleansing the wound, leaving the left hand for lifting and applying the dressing on to the wound. Both hands may be used, making sure the gloved hands do not touch the patient's skin.

8.9
Paediatric preoperative nursing care

See also Procedures 3.13 and 3.14.

Psychological preparation
Small children do not experience fear of operation, anaesthesia and possible death, which are natural typical fears of adults. Their greatest fears are separation from parents, unfamiliar environment and inability to understand the reasons for hunger and the strange activities around them.

Anxiety is often revealed in the frequent questioning of the older child who is apprehensive, but simple truthful explanation is invariably accepted if all the preoperative preparations are directed towards 'getting him/her better.'

Introduction to such pieces of equipment as oxygen tents and monitors are important and worthwhile in achieving postoperative cooperation, as is preoperative physiotherapy in cases where this will be necessary postoperatively.

In cases of elective surgery visits from the anaesthetist and/or members of the theatre team can also be helpful, especially to the parents who must be kept fully in the picture at all times and who will require to sign the consent form after the surgeon has discussed the planned treatment with them.

Whenever possible parents should be allowed to go to the reception area of the theatre suite and if suitable they should be present when their child comes round from the anaesthetic.

Physical preparation

1   The child's current weight should be recorded on the medicine prescription sheet.

2   A urine specimen should be obtained and routine tests carried out.

3   Routine bowel preparation is not required unless it is known that the child is constipated or bowel surgery is planned.

4   Children having general anaesthesia should have nothing to eat or drink for a minimum of 5 hours prior to planned onset of surgery. They should be given a 30% glucose drink between 12 midnight and 3 a.m. (for an 8–9 a.m. theatre start).

It is a pity to waken a child at 3 a.m. if he/she has been awake between 12 midnight and 3 a.m. but there is a danger of depleting the liver of glycogen store when giving an anaesthetic to a child who has been without nourishment for too long. Therefore if the child has slept until 3 a.m. he/she should be gently wakened and given the 30% glucose drink with nothing by mouth after that (see item 1 Immediate preparation).

5   The child should be bathed prior to operation, paying particular attention to finger and toe nails, umbilicus and ears. Talcum powder should be avoided. The child's hair should be washed, if necessary.

Immediate preparation

1   If the child has medicines prescribed check with anaesthetist to see if he/she wishes these to be administered (e.g. 6 a.m. medicines). Medicines may be made up in relatively small quantities of fluid and can be safely administered, if necessary. It is often important to maintain the blood levels of the medicine concerned.

2 The child should be dressed in an open-back operation gown and hair covered with a disposable paper cap.

3 The child should be encouraged to pass urine before leaving the ward, but at all events the nurse accompanying the child to the theatre should know when he/she last passed urine.

If the child is unable to pass urine either in the ward area or in the theatre reception area the nurse must inform the theatre staff before the child is actually taken into the theatre. This is particularly important when abdominal surgery is planned. The surgeon may request catheterisation. It is also important, whatever type of surgery is planned because once the child is anaesthetised he/she will relax and possibly be incontinent, thus contaminating the sterile field.

4 The nurse accompanying the child to the theatre should be the child's 'own nurse' or one with whom he/she is familiar. The nurse should know all the relevant details about the child including diagnosis and, if possible what operation is planned with particular reference to the site, e.g. *left* inguinal hernia.

5 Other specific preoperative procedures, e.g. cross-matching of blood, haemoglobin estimation will be arranged by the medical staff.

8

8.10
Paediatric postoperative nursing care

See also Procedure 3.15.

Immediate postoperative care

1   The child will almost certainly be nursed by suitably trained and experienced nurses in the recovery area of the theatre suite. The child will be transferred to the ward, when the anaesthetist is satisfied that recovery from the anaesthetic is complete. The child, accompanied by a trained nurse and a porter, should be transferred in a lateral position with a good airway maintained by forward support of the jaw (this directs the child's tongue away from the air passages).

2   The child is received into a quiet ward and if fully conscious is allowed one pillow and encouraged to sleep.

3   Close observation of the following is necessary:
   colour
   pulse and respiration rates
   operation site
   fluid balance

The child's vital signs recordings should be charted as directed (usually hourly initially).

Continuing care

1   Restlessness and pain should be dealt with by repositioning, reassurance and analgesics as prescribed.

2   If vomiting is troublesome an anti-emetic may be prescribed by the doctor.

3 The first postoperative urine voided **must always be recorded** in the nursing Kardex.

4 As the child recovers a second pillow should be given, if necessary. Further pillows may be added until the upright position is reached.

5 The child is sponged down and changed out of the operation gown, his/her hair combed and the bed made comfortable.

6 Fluids should never be withheld from a child (unless on medical instructions) once the swallowing reflex has returned. If vomiting is a problem, it should be reported and dealt with as mentioned in item 2.

7 There are many children who, after minor surgery, are hungry and will enjoy a light meal by afternoon or evening.

8 Early ambulation is encouraged in most instances, but is rarely a problem with children.

Reporting

The nurse returning from the theatre should be able to give the rest of the nursing staff a description of what has been done at the operation and any special instructions she/he may have been given. A theatre card giving details of, for example, drainage tubes may also accompany the child on return from the theatre.

The medicine prescription sheet suitably written up with postoperative medication (sedation/analgesic) should always accompany the child on return from the theatre.

It should always be remembered that no matter how minor the surgery, it is a very worrying time for the child's relatives. Time should be spent in giving as much information as possible to the parents and they should have free access to their child wherever possible, to allay these fears. More detailed postoperative care will be explained to individual requirements, e.g. intravenous therapy, dressings.

8

8.11
Humidification therapy—croupette and humidaire tents

Humidification is used to:
  loosen viscid secretions of the respiratory passages
  assist expectoration of viscid secretions from the respiratory passages
  provide a soothing effect on the respiratory passages

Equipment
Croupette or humidaire frame and canopy
Diapump or air compressor or piped air
Pressure tubing
Distilled water and jar
Ice in a receiver
Air-temperature thermometer

Preparation of the tent
1 Erect the tent according to the manufacturers' instructions.
2 Fill the water jar with distilled water to the appropriate level. Attach atomiser.
3 Put ice in the ice-box, if necessary.

Preparation of the child
Minimal clothing and bed covers, (nappy or pants only).
Support the child in the upright position (unless contraindicated).
Help the child to overcome apprehension by playing

with the child and introduce a **safe toy** into the tent.

Continuing care of the equipment

1   Check pressure dial and appearance of water vapour.

2   Check water jar—refilled with distilled water, as required.

3   Check temperature in the tent (**must not exceed 21°C**).

4   Ice-box replenished, as necessary.

5   Wipe inside of canopy frequently to ensure an unobstructed view of the child.

6   Check atomiser for sediment on the filter.

8.12
Oxygen therapy with tents

Equipment
As per Procedure 8.11 with the addition of:
Oxygen tubing
Oxygen atomiser (if long-term oxygen therapy is
  required)

Preparation of the equipment
1   Prepare tent as per Procedure 8.11.
2   Attach oxygen tubing either:
  to nozzle on distilled water jar for oxygen of low
  humidity
     OR
  to oxygen inlet on back of tent for oxygen of
  high humidity
3   Before use, the fine adjustments for oxygen flow
must be opened before the main tap is turned on.
The tent is flushed first with oxygen before the rate
of flow is regulated to that prescribed by the doctor.

Preparation of the child
As per Procedure 8.11.

Care of the child during the procedure
1   Remain within the view of the child in order to
overcome his/her feelings of loneliness.
2   Assess the child's general condition at regular
intervals.
3   Ensure frequent change of clothing.
4   Ensure frequent nasopharyngeal suction.
5   Ensure adequate intake of fluid and check
output.

8

287

6 Observe:
     restlessness, irritability of the child
     child's colour—flushed, pale or cyanosed
     record TPR frequently as instructed

Special dangers and precautions

No nylon clothes.

No friction toys.

All electrical apparatus, for example, suction mach-
     ine, diapump should be maintained regularly and
     left switched off when not in use.

No electrical apparatus inside the tent.

Prevent overheating inside the tent by use of ice.

Keep thermometer out of the child's reach.

Aftercare of the child and the equipment

Dismantle and clean the tent according to the manu-
     facturer's instructions. Ensure warmth and com-
     fort for the child and report on his/her general
     condition to the nurse in charge.

   NOTE. Many small children can be nursed naked
in the croupette especially if they are febrile. In this
instance it is necessary to reassure the parents.

8.13
Jejunal biopsy using a Crosby capsule

A Crosby capsule is used to obtain a specimen of jejunal mucosa to aid in the diagnosis of malabsorption (see Procedure 3.46). It is carried out by a doctor in the X-ray department and should be initiated, if possible, in the treatment room. Sedation may be prescribed prior to procedure.

Equipment
Crosby capsule
20 ml syringe
Gauze swabs
Water for lubrication in gallipot
Adhesive tape
Undiluted Delrosa in a gallipot (cup of juice available)
Vomit bowl
Universal container with normal saline (0·9%). If an antispasmodic medicine is prescribed for administration during the procedure appropriate equipment is required
Medicine prescription and recording sheet

Preparation of the child
1   The procedure **must be explained** to the child, as simply as possible and reassurance throughout the procedure must be given. If the parents are to be present during the procedure they too must understand the procedure.

8

2   Written permission of parent/guardian **must be obtained.**
3   The child is fasted overnight.
4   Sedation given prior to the procedure as prescribed.
5   Small children should have double thickness tubegauze mitts put on to prevent them tampering with the tube.
6   Until the tube is successfully passed, the child should be firmly wrapped in a blanket.

Procedure
1   The Crosby capsule is lubricated and passed orally by the doctor until the appropriate mark on the tube is reached. The free end of the tube is securely taped to the child's gown or cheek. The antispasmodic medicine may then be administered as prescribed.
2   The child is then nursed on his/her right side in order to encourage peristaltic movement of the tube through the pylorus (approximately 1 hour). From time to time the tube may be advanced and check X-ray films taken until the Crosby capsule reaches the correct position.
3   The trigger is then 'fired' by the doctor (using the 20 ml syringe) and the capsule is carefully withdrawn (see Procedure 3.46, items 5–7).
4   The specimen is removed from the Crosby capsule, placed in a universal container containing saline (labelled appropriately) and sent to the laboratory as soon as possible with the appropriate form.

Aftercare of the child
1   On return to the ward the child is made comfortable, given a drink and reassured.

2   The child's pulse and respiration rates are recorded hourly or as per medical instructions.

3   The child is observed for bleeding.

Aftercare of the Crosby capsule
See Procedure 3.46.

9
Psychiatric Nursing Procedures

9

9.1
Electroconvulsive therapy (ECT)

Electroconvulsive therapy is an impirical form of treatment which is used mainly in the treatment of depression, particularly the endogenous type. However, it may also be used in:

mania—not quite so common and must be given more frequently

schizophrenia—where there is an affective disorder or catatonic stupor

epilepsy—rarely, but sometimes in the case of psychomotor epilepsy

Contraindications
During pregnancy
6 to 8 weeks postnatal—danger of embolism
Recent fractures
Recent cardiac infarction
Respiratory infections
Active tuberculosis
Organic brain disease, e.g. tumour, dementia

Early preparation of the patient
1   The patient is given a full physical examination, including chest X-ray. The result of the physical examination is recorded on the consent form by the doctor together with the patient's age, weight, blood pressure and current medication.
2   The patient is prepared psychologically by the doctor, i.e. an explanation is given and the patient's fears allayed. This is also recorded on the consent form by the doctor.

3   Laterality test is carried out and recorded by the doctor.

4   The patient, ideally signs the consent form but, due to inability by the patient, the nearest relative or guardian may sign the consent form.

Immediate preparation of the patient

1   The patient is fasted from midnight.

2   Night sedation is kept to a minimum.

3   **On the morning of treatment** the patient's temperature, pulse and respiration are taken and recorded on the consent form. No medicines are given unless specially prescribed. The patient requires to be strictly observed in order that he/she does not deliberately eat or drink. Should this happen, the treatment must be cancelled.

4   The patient is requested to empty his/her urinary bladder and bowels.

5   The patient's dentures are removed. No jewellery, hair-pins etc., or cosmetics should be worn.

6   The patient is dressed in light, non-constricting clothes, e.g. pyjamas/nightdress, dressing gown and slippers—no stocking or socks are worn.

7   The patient may either walk to the treatment room or be taken by trolley or bed. In the latter case, the patient should be covered with a warm light blanket.

8   Relevant charts and the consent form must accompany the patient to the treatment room.

9   An admission bed is prepared for the patient's return.

Equipment

Trolley containing:

Top shelf:

Ampoules of

(a) sodium thiopentone or Brietal (anaesthetic)

(b) Brevidal E. or Scoline (muscle relaxant)
(c) distilled water
(d) atropine sulphate 0.6 mg
Selection of syringes, e.g. 20 ml, 10 ml and 5 ml
Selection of needles including butterfly needles
Bowl containing Ectrononlyte solution
Gallipot containing Teepol 25% in spirit
Laryngoscope
Mouth gags
Airways
Gauze swabs
Disposal bag
Bottom shelf:
Emergency box containing medicines and resusci-
  tation equipment
And:
Oxygen
Suction apparatus
ECT machine and electrodes (electrodes covered
  with recommended pads)
Defibrillator

Procedure
1   The patient lies flat on the treatment trolley,
covered with a treatment blanket and his/her head
supported by one pillow.
2   An anaesthetist, a doctor and two nurses participate in the treatment.
3   If necessary the anaesthetist will administer
atropine sulphate 0.6 mg intravenously and record.
4   The anaesthetist administers the anaesthetic,
muscle relaxant and oxygen.
5   The patient's feet are exposed for observation
when the shock is administered.
6   The doctor carried out the ECT. When the

shock is administered the patient will have a modified grand mal seizure.

7   During the seizure, **one nurse lightly holds** the patient's arms across his/her chest while **the second nurse lightly holds** the patient's lower abdomen and legs.

8   When the anaesthetist is satisfied that the patient is fully recovered and is breathing spontaneously, he/she is taken back to the ward.

9   On return to the ward the patient is placed in bed in a lateral position (see Procedure 3.15, Post-operative care—general notes).

Continuing patient care

1   Maintain a clear airway.

2   Check the patient's pulse and respiration rates frequently.

3   Note headache, amnesia and confusion and their duration.

4   When the patient has fully recovered from the effects of the anaesthetic provide him/her with a light meal.

5   Note any changes in the patient's affect (mood) and general activities.

NOTE. Analgesic may be prescribed by the doctor for severe post electroconvulsive therapy headache.

If unilateral electroconvulsive therapy is being used, the electrodes are placed over the non-dominant hemisphere of the brain. It is therefore important to establish whether the patient is right-handed or left-handed in order to ascertain which is the non-dominant hemisphere. This information **must be clearly** registered on the laterality chart. If there is no clearly defined dominant hemisphere bi-lateral electroconvulsive therapy is given.

9.2
Modified insulin therapy

Modified insulin therapy is a method of treatment which is used in an effort to promote appetite and so aid relaxation where there has been recent weight loss due to neurotic illness. This form of treatment would appear to be used infrequently.

NOTE. To eliminate the possibility of diabetes mellitus urine and blood sugar tests are **essential**.

Preparation of the patient
The procedure is explained to the patient and his/ her fears allayed.
The patient is fasted overnight.
The patient is weighed.

Procedure
1 At 7 a.m. the patient is given a subcutaneous injection of prescribed soluble insulin
Dosage. On the first day the patient is given 10 units, thereafter this dosage is increased daily by 5 to 10 units, to 40 or more units, according to the response. **The response** being that the patient is only allowed to develop **mild** hypoglycaemic signs and symptoms.
2 The patient is nursed in absorbent sheet and nightwear. The environment is kept quiet and the patient is encouraged to relax and drowse.
3 The patient is kept under **constant nursing observation** and the pulse and respiration rates are recorded every 15 minutes.
4 After $2\frac{1}{2}$ to 3 hours following the injection of

insulin the patient is roused and given a glucose drink followed by a breakfast of about 4000 kJ containing 20 to 25 g of protein. This breakfast must be appetising and the patient should be encouraged to eat it all.

5   After breakfast the patient may be allowed up and about and it should be seen that he/she takes the other meals properly.

6   In the afternoon the patient may become slightly hypoglycaemic (the patient must be informed of this). The symptoms can be relieved by eating sweets or taking a drink of sweetened tea or fruit juice.

7   The patient's weight should be recorded at the beginning and at the end of the course of treatment, as well as weekly during the treatment.

8   The treatment is usually continued for a few weeks until the patient attains his/her normal weight.

Danger

The danger is that the patient may, while hypoglycaemic, drift into a coma.

NOTES. *Symptoms of hypoglycaemia:* feelings of weakness, emptiness, shakiness, faintness and hunger.

Signs of hypoglycaemia: alteration in the pulse rate, sweating and tremor.

Instead of becoming drowsy the patient may become restless, disinhibited, laughing or crying.

If there is muscular twitching or the patient becomes not easily rousable the treatment must be interrupted **at once** by the oral or intravenous administration of glucose or the subcutaneous administration of 0.5 ml of 1 in 1000 (0.1%) adrenaline. Therefore an **emergency tray** for this eventuality

must be at hand. If the treatment has to be interrupted in this way, the morning dose of insulin is
usually subsequently reduced by at least 10 units by
the doctor.

9

9.3
Monoamine oxidase inhibitor therapy

Monoamine oxidase inhibitor (MAOI) medicines, e.g. phenelzine (Nardil) are sometimes prescribed in the treatment of psychotic depression. Inpatients are treated with these medicines.

Danger
As a result of administration of monoamine oxidase inhibitors tyramine remains unoxidased and, being a pressor amine, it produces severe clinical effects when taken in conjunction with food and drink of a high tyramine content. Large doses of the pressor amine build up in the body and it has been known to cause a *hypertensive crisis* with severe headache, cerebral haemorrhage and death.

Strictly forbidden food and drink
Cheese—all kinds—raw, cooked or processed
Yeast and meat extracts—Oxo, Bovril, Marmite
Pickled herring
Broad bean pods
Liver paté
Bananas
Chianti wine and alcohol in general

Food and drink which may be taken in moderation

Chicken liver	Beef liver	Liquorice
Yoghurt	Creams	Tinned milk
Chocolate	Cola	Complan
Coffee	Figs	Avocado pears

Proprietary cough and cold medicines

These foods and drinks may cause symptoms in some patients.

NOTES. Monoamine oxidase inhibitors can increase the action of other medicines such as:

Anti-Parkinsons	Pressor medicines
Amphetamines	Morphine
Barbiturates	Tricyclic antidepressants
Pethidine	

A toxic reaction may follow their combined use.

In order to eliminate the possibility of severe toxic reactions when monoamine oxidase inhibitor medicines are used the doctor and the nurse have certain responsibilities.

Doctor's responsibilities

To ascertain the patient's recent medicine treatment, especially within the 3 previous weeks, before prescribing a monoamine oxidase inhibitor.

To allow 2–3 weeks to elapse before prescribing another antidepressant medicine (especially a tricyclic antidepressant) after a recent course of monoamine oxidase inhibitor therapy.

To explain to the patient the dangers of consuming the prohibited foods and drink while on monoamine oxidase inhibitor therapy.

Nurse's responsibilities

To ensure that none of the prohibited foods or drink are consumed by the patient.

To observe the patient and **report any side effects,** especially palpitations, sweating, flushes and severe headache **(these must be reported to the doctor immediately).**

To obtain a treatment card for the patient and to give instructions to the patient:

(a) to carry the treatment card at all times and, on

discharge, to present it to his/her own doctor, especially if still on monoamine oxidase inhibitor therapy or has been within the past 3 weeks, and (b) to report any side effects immediately to the medical or nursing staff.

NOTE. Should a hypertensive crisis develop, it may be controlled by the administration of Pentolinium or Metaraminol which should be available in the *emergency box*.

9.4
Treatment of alcoholism by Antabuse 200

The aim of treating alcoholism by Antabuse 200 is that the medicine will act as a deterrent and, therefore, support the patient in his/her refusal of alcohol. Having experienced (or been told) the results of combining the two, it is hoped that he/she will not wish to risk these consequences.

Antabuse 200 interferes with the normal oxidation of alcohol and in so doing causes an excess of acetaldehyde in the body. It is the acetaldehyde poisoning that produces the symptoms upon whose discouraging effect the treatment depends.

Abstem has a similar action but less severe.

Procedure

1 The doctor determines that the patient is reasonably physically fit.

NOTE. *Contraindications* are cardiac decompensation and severe kidney or liver damage. These are an absolute bar to treatment.

2 The patient must be willing to participate and cooperate with this form of treatment. The treatment is fully explained to the patient.

NOTE. Not all patients who commence this form of medicine treatment undertake the test dose reaction (alcohol).

3 The medicine is administered as follows:

Day 1—800 mg
  2—600 mg
  3—400 mg

4—200 mg
5—200 mg

Subsequently, 200 mg or 100 mg are given daily until otherwise prescribed by the doctor.

4   After 5 days on the medicine, a test dose (10–15 ml) of alcohol may be given to the patient (patient's normal choice of alcohol).

NOTE. **It is extremely important** that the patient is in bed when experiencing the reaction and that resuscitation equipment including medicines are on hand should severe reaction occur, thus warranting medical intervention.

5   Continuous observation of the patient, including recording of pulse rate and blood pressure is maintained throughout the reaction time.

6   Within 20 minutes of taking the alcohol the patient will develop a highly unpleasant reaction:

intense flushing of the face, neck and upper chest
tachycardia and palpitations
headache
dyspnoea
nausea and vomiting

7   If, however, the initial reaction is not marked, a further 10–15 ml of alcohol may be given to the patient.

8   If a reaction is too severe, it can be interrupted by the intravenous administration of ascorbic acid by the doctor.

9   The patient should be advised to avoid:

all foods containing malt vinegar, wine vinegar or sauces and pickles made with fermented vinegar, since these contain alcohol
the use of alcohol based toiletries such as cologne or after-shave
cough syrups and tonics containing alcohol

NOTE   Antabuse 200 potentiates the action of

barbiturates, monoamine oxidase inhibitors, paraldehyde, phenytoin and any other medicines which are metabolised by oxidation.

It is rapidly absorbed from the gastrointestinal tract and although it is of low toxicity, it is slowly excreted and can be detected in body fluids up to 7 days after cessation of treatment.

Follow up

All patients who are prescribed Antabuse 200 should be issued with an ANTABUSE 200 WARNING CARD which outlines the dangers should he/she contemplate, at any time, taking alcohol whilst on treatment.

9

10
Chemotherapy and Radiotherapy Nursing Procedures

10

10.1
Nursing care of patients receiving cytotoxic chemotherapy

Cytotoxic chemotherapy is a drug therapy used to effect a remission or cure of a malignant disease or condition.

Equipment
Appropriate to the route of administration of the cytotoxic drugs:
Oral administration
Intramuscular administration
Intravenous administration
Intra-arterial administration
Intracavitary administration

Preparation of patient
Explain the procedure to the patient and provide psychological reassurance and emotional support.
Record the patient's weight and height.
Order an appropriate and light diet for the patient.
    NOTE. A wig may be ordered for the patient, if necessary.

10

Nursing care and observation of the patient
1   Encourage the patient to rest.
2   The patient must have a minimum oral intake of 2 litres of fluid per day. Observe for signs of dehydration.
3   Give the patient frequent and regular mouth care.

4 Record the patient's urinary output and note any dysuria and frequency.

5 Note any alteration in the patient's bowel habit, i.e. constipation or diarrhoea.

6 Observe the patient's skin for any skin rashes.

7 Observe and note any alteration in the patient's mood and behaviour especially depression.

8 Observe intravenous/intra-arterial needle site for local extravasation.

9 Observe and note any alopecia.

10 Report if the patient complains of tumour pain or tingling fingers.

11 Observe the patient for anaphylaxis or hypoglycaemia.

12 Observe the patient for any signs of infection, e.g. sore throat.

Cytotoxic and other medicines

Actinomycin D and Adriamycin can cause myocardial toxicity. The patient has an electrocardiograph (ECG) before these are administered. These normally cause the urine to be red in colour.

Aspirin or salycilic compounds are never given to the patient after cytotoxic chemotherapy because they can cause internal bleeding.

Bleomycin is mixed with 1 ml of lignocaine plain when administered intramuscularly to afford the patient minimum of discomfort. Tumour pain can occur after the administration of Bleomycin.

Cyclophosphamide: the patient may flush facially when cyclophosphamide is administered intravenously or intra-arterially. It must be stored in a refrigerator otherwise it loses its potency.

Natulan is a monoamine oxidase inhibitor (MAOI) and therefore the patient must receive an appropriate diet (see Procedure 9.3).

Methotrexate causes mouth ulceration. It is incompatible with sulphonamide.

Vinblastine and Vincristine can cause local extravasation of the needle site when administered intravenously or intra-arterially. Neurotoxicity to Vincristine is often indicated by the patient complaining of tingling of the fingers. This must be reported to the doctor.

NOTES. After cytotoxic chemotherapy the patient's bone marrow is depressed and as a result he/she is more **prone to infection**.

Nurses must be aware of the storage requirements of cytotoxic agents, e.g. see *cyclophosphamide*.

Nurses must be aware of the side-effect and incompatibilities of cytotoxic agents, e.g. see *Methotrexate*.

10

10.2
Skin care of patients receiving radiotherapy

Radiotherapy is the irradiation treatment of non-malignant and malignant diseases and conditions. It is used to effect a remission or cure of the disease or condition.

Equipment
60 kV (superficial) x-ray machine
125 kV (ipac) x-ray machine
300 kV (conventional) x-ray machine
4 MeV (linear accelerator) x-ray machine

Care of the patient's skin during treatment
Treatment by superficial, ipac or conventional machines. The skin of the treatment areas should be kept dry and pen marks must be left on.

Treatment by linear accelerator. The skin of the treatment areas is usually 'tattooed' and the patient can wash the skin of the treatment areas. **Only when** the patient receiving such treatment has a **wax build up** at the time of treatment will he/she **not be allowed** to wash the skin of the treatment areas.

Metal based ointments, talcs or soaps. No metal based ointments, talcs or soaps must be used during the coarse of treatment on the skin of the treatment areas. Purified talcum or Johnson's Baby Powder should be applied 3 times per day to the skin of the treatment areas.

10

Washing treatment area skin. The patient allowed to wash the skin treatment areas **should not use** soap or rub dry with a towel. The areas should be dabbed dry using cotton wool.

Shaving. The male patient receiving radiotherapy to his face or neck should electric shave only.

Clothing. The patient should wear loose cotton garments next to the skin.

Perfume, after-shave, etc. Deodorants, perfumes and after-shaves must not be applied to the skin of the treatment areas.

Do not allow the patient to expose his/her treatment areas to the sun, cold winds or rain.

Observing and reporting skin reactions

Erythema—reddening of the skin of the treatment areas. Normally occurs towards the end of the treatment course.

Dry desquamation—the skin of the treatment areas becomes dry, cracked and scaly.

Moist desquamation—moist ulcers develop in the skin of the treatment areas.

NOTES. Report any skin changes to the doctor and to the radiographer in the radiotherapy treatment centre.

Skin reactions occur quicker in the groins and axillae therefore good nursing observation is required.

10

Mouth care of patient receiving radiotherapy to the mouth

Sodium bicarbonate solution should be used to clean the patient's mouth and he/she should have hourly mouth washes. Glycerine of thymol **must not be used**.

The patient's mouth must be observed for any sign of infection and the doctor informed.

If a reaction starts in the patient's mouth and he/she wears dentures encourage him/her to wear the dentures only at meal times.

Dressings to skin areas receiving radio-theraphy

Apply 'Melolin' to irradiated skin areas.

Use small amounts of prescribed aqueous solution to clean skin or fungating tissue within the treatment areas.

Infected fungating masses—Milton 1 in 200 (0.5%) wicks can be used.

Dressings must only be retained in position with Micropore or Netalast. **Do not use** zinc oxide or adhesive tape.

NOTE. *Sutures* in the area treated by radiotherapy remain in situ until the tenth postoperative day.

Eye pads are applied for 4 hours after radiotherapy to the inner canthus or eye. Prescribed eye drops are used prior to radiotherapy treatment.

10

11
X-ray Procedures and Notes

11

11.1
Preparation and care of patient for x-ray examinations—general notes

Ensure that an explanation is given to the patient prior to the x-ray examination.

If a general anaesthetic is required preoperative and postoperative care appropriate to the x-ray examination must be carried out (see Procedures 3.13, 3.14 and 3.15).

The patient should wear x-ray gown. (In the case of out-patients such gowns are supplied in the x-ray department.)

Previous x-rays must always accompany the patient to the x-ray department.

Code of practice. Any nurse who accompanies a patient to the x-ray department and is present during x-ray procedures requires to comply with *Code of Practice for the Protection of Persons against Ionising Radiations* operational in the department.

Medicine kardex must accompany the patient to the x-ray department when a general anaesthetic is being given and when a percutaneous transhepatic cholangiography is being done.

11

11.2
Preparation and care of patients for x-ray examination—specific notes

Air encephalogram
Prepare the patient as for general anaesthetic (see Procedure 11.1).

After x-ray examination return the patient to bed and place him/her in a recumbent position.

NOTES. 'Narcan' must be available should respiratory failure occur following the administration of 'Operdine' and 'Dropleptan' (which are given to sedate the patient).

Severe headache usually follows an air encephalogram.

Barium enema
The patient can have a light breakfast on the morning of examination (tea and toast). No solid food thereafter.

Bowel preparation is usually carried out in the x-ray department unless the ward nursing staff are requested to do so.

The examination will take 3 to 4 hours.

The patient is encouraged to take fluids to prevent constipation after procedure. An aperient may be prescribed.

Barium meal
The patient must have nothing to eat or drink after 10.00 p.m. on the night before the examination.

The initial examination takes approximately 1 hour.

The patient is encouraged to take fluids to prevent constipation after procedure. An aperient may be prescribed.

Cardiac catheterisation

Prior to the procedure As the femoral artery is usually used for cardiac catheterisation, a pubic shave is routinely carried out in the ward. If the patient's arm requires to be shaved as an alternate site this is carried out in the x-ray department.

After the procedure. The patient is returned to bed and the following nursing observations are carried out, initially every 15 minutes, then as required.

Puncture site for bleeding. If bleeding occurs apply direct pressure over the puncture site and notify the doctor.

The limb distal to the puncture site for colour, sensation and pulse.

Blood pressure.

The patient should be confined to bed for 24 hours with legs straight.

Carotid angiography

Prepare the patient as for general anaesthetic (see Procedure 11.1).

After x-ray examination return the patient to bed.

Check puncture site for bleeding every 15 minutes for 2 hours. If bleeding occurs apply direct pressure over the puncture site and notify the doctor.

Bleeding may occur obstructing patient's airways.

Cholecystography

The examination will take approximately 2 hours in two or more stages and will occupy a part of 2 days.

PART I: no specific preparation of the patient is required.

11

PART II: the patient takes all the supplied Telepaque tablets (total six) with water, one at a time. **Do not crush the tablets.** After the tablets have been taken no more food must be taken by the patient. Fat-containing drinks must be avoided, e.g. milk (even in tea).

Excretion urography (intravenous pyelography—IVP)
No specific preparation of the patient is required for an excretion urography.

Aorta-arteriography
Prepare the patient as for general anaesthetic (see Procedure 11.1).

The patient is bathed and pubic area is shaved

After the x-ray examination the patient is returned to bed for 24 hours.

Check puncture site for bleeding every 15 minutes for 2 hours. If bleeding occurs apply direct pressure over the femoral artery at the site of the puncture and notify the doctor.

Intravenous cholangiography
No specific preparation of the patient is required for an intravenous cholangiography.

Myelography
The patient may have a light meal prior to the examination.

After the x-ray examination the patient is returned to bed.

NOTES. If Myodil is used **avoid** lowering the patient's head to prevent Myodil entering the skull.

If 'Amipaque' is used care as for lumber puncture.

11

Pacing catheter
The patient's chest and shoulder should be shaved, if appropriate. Patient is fasted from 10.00 p.m. the night prior to procedure.

Translumber aorto-arteriography
Prepare the patient as for general anaesthetic (see Procedure 11.1).

After the x-ray examination the patient is returned to bed.

Check the patient's pulse and blood pressure every 15 minutes for 2 hours.

Small bowel barium enema
1   Fast the patient from 10.00 p.m. the night prior to procedure.

2   Naso/duodenal tube is passed in either Clinical Measurement department or X-Ray department prior to examination.

3   The examination will take 1–2 hours.

4   Fluids are encouraged to prevent constipation after the procedure. An aperient may be prescribed.

Lymphangiography
1   The contrast medium includes a blue dye which shows through the lymphatics of the feet. This may show in the patient's skin and urine.

2   X-ray films are taken on injection of the contrast medium and 24 hours later.

Venography
Usually no specific preparation but the patient should be informed of possible discomfort during the procedure. If a femoral venography is carried out preparation is as for aorto-arteriography (see page 322).

11

11.3
Veripaque enema

A veripaque enema is normally carried out in the x-ray department but may be carried out in the ward, as requested.

Equipment
Trolley with:
St Bartholomew's barium catheter
Veripaque
Enema bag
50 ml syringe
Connection
KY jelly or lubricant
Spigot
Gate clip (tube clip)
Lotion thermometer
Jug for tepid water (30°C)
Gauze swabs
Disposable glove
Disposal bag

Preparation of equipment
1   Mix one vial of Veripaque in 1 litre of tepid water (30°C) at least 10 minutes before use and shake well.
2   Fill enema bag with the Veripaque solution and run the fluid through the tube to the connection and clamp with the gate clip (tube clip).

Preparation of the patient
Explain the procedure to the patient and gain his/

her cooperation (see Procedure 11.2, Barium enema).

Procedure
1   As per Procedure 3.7, items 1–3 inclusive.
2   Using the disposable glove insert KY jelly just in and around the patient's anus.
3   Lubricate the catheter and gently insert into the patient's rectum for 10–13 cm.
4   Inflate the catheter balloon using the syringe piston drawn back to 30 ml mark. Withdraw syringe and spigot the small air tube at the side of the catheter.
5   Connect up enema bag and control the flow of the Veripaque with the gate clip (tube clip).

NOTES. Once the enema has been administered and the catheter removed **instruct the patient to rock his/her knees from side to side**—this distributes the Veripaque around the patient's bowel.

The patient will experience abdominal pains some of which may be spasmodic (likened to labour contractions). These pains will become more and more frequent until they become continuous and the patient just has to go to the toilet. **It is important to encourage** the patient to retain the enema solution until this point has been reached.

When the patient has completed his/her toilet give him/her a cup of tea or coffee plus a biscuit and put him/her back to bed. Encourage the patient to try going to the toilet at least twice more, once just before the examination.

6   Clear away equipment, make the patient comfortable and unscreen the bed.

Aftercare of equipment
If a bedpan is used: as per Procedure 1.19.
If a commode is used: as per Procedure 1.21.

11

Observation and reporting
As per Procedure 1.18.

Nursing notes
It is necessary that the patient rests for about 1 hour following the enema to allow the bowel to stop contracting.

Patients for double contrast enemas require to be weighed before x-ray examination begins.

11

11.4
Preparation of the patient for ultrasonic examination

Aorta; kidney; liver; pancreas; spleen
The patient has nothing by mouth except water 8 hours before the examination. No carbonated or fizzy drinks.

Pelvis, lower abdomen
The patient's urinary bladder must be filled. He/she should be encouraged to have plenty to drink for a few hours before the examination and not to pass any urine.

Gall bladder
As for cholecystogram including contrast medium (see Procedure 11.2).

Thyroid
No specific preparation of the patient is required.

11

12
Administration of Medicines

12

12.1
Administration of oral medicines

Equipment
Trolley containing:
All medicines required
Graduated medicine glasses
Standard 5 ml medicine spoons
Jug of cold water
Small tray or plate for carrying medicines to the patient's bedside
Receiver for used spoons and glasses
Medical wipes
Medicine prescription and recording sheets

NOTES
1   **Always** have two nurses giving medicines, one in a checking or supervising capacity.
2   **Never** leave the trolley unattended. **Always** lock the trolley if called away in an emergency.
3   Identify the name of the patient with the name on the medicine prescription sheet and the patient's identity wrist band and any other checking system.
4   Check the medicine sensitivity column.
5   Read the prescription carefully. It should be printed legibly; metric system used; prescribed and signed by a registered medical practitioner.
6   Select the medicine and check the label with the prescription. Check expiry date.
7   Ensure that the label is kept clean (if liquid medicine) by holding the bottle with the label uppermost against the palm of the pouring hand.

12

8 Shake all medicines well, particularly antibiotics in suspension.

9 Hold the medicine glass at eye level while pouring the medicine.

10 When administering tablets or capsules, shake the number required on to the lid of the container and from there on to a spoon to avoid touching them.

11 When giving powders, place on a spoon and then on the back of the patient's tongue or mix with water.

12 Give tooth-staining medicines with a straw.

13 Give effervescent tablets (with water) or as prescribed.

4 Glass medicine glasses are **not used** to administer medicine to children, psychiatric and mentally handicapped patients.

Administration

1 Check the identity of the patient.

2 Give medicines at the time ordered and give before or after meals as instructed.

3 Make unpleasant medicines as agreeable as possible by following their administration with a sweet or drink of fruit juice, if this is allowed.

4 Stay with the patient until he/she takes the medicine. **Do not** leave the medicines on the patient's bedside locker.

5 Note administration (non-administration) on medicine recording sheet.

6 Controlled medicines are recorded in the controlled medicine record book in the ward.

7 Medicine keys should remain on person of nurse in charge of the ward or senior nurse administering medicines.

12

12.2
Injections

Types
Intramuscular: most common route for the injection of medicines. Medicine injected deeply into the body of a muscle.
Hypodermic or subcutaneous: less commonly used except for the injection of *insulin*.
Intradermal: done by the doctor.

Equipment
Basic equipment is the same for all types of injections:

Foil tray

Syringe }
Needles } prepacked

Medicine either in ampoule or multidose container

Ampoule of sterile water is sometimes required to dissolve a medicine in powder form

File (may be necessary to break some glass ampoules)

2 or 3 isopropyl alcohol prepared swabs (e.g. Mediswab)

Medicine prescription sheet stating:
  name of patient
  medicine to be administered, its dosage (and strength)
  route of administration
  time of administration

Disposal bag for waste materials

NOTE. Replace syringe and needles in the foil tray and dispose of in appropriate containers.

Preparation of injection

1   Check name of medicine with patient's medicine prescription sheet details between two nurses, one of whom **must be** trained.

2   Wash hands.

3   Open packs and assemble the syringe and needle, observing strict asepsis throughout.

4   Carefully break open ampoule protecting fingers with appropriate size of Isopropyl swab around ampoule top. If difficult to break, file slightly. Draw up the medicine into the syringe. Expel air bubbles in the syringe back into the ampoule and **not** into the atmosphere.

OR

Swab the top of the multidose container with isopropyl swabs, insert needle, inject air from the syringe into the container, then draw up slightly more than required amount of the medicine into the syringe. Tilt container upwards and expel air bubbles and excess medicine back into the container.

5   Remove the needle from the container or ampoule cover carefully with the protective sheath and place the syringe on the foil tray.

6   Again carefully check the medicine with the patient's name and details with the medicine prescription sheet.

7   Go to the patient and identify by his/her identity wristband or verbally or both.

8   Explain the nature of the procedure to the patient.

9   Ensure privacy.

10   Clean the area of injection site with prepared swab.

11   Insert needle approximately three-quarters of its length, at an appropriate angle. Withdraw piston

gently to ensure the needle is not in a blood vessel. Then slowly but firmly give the injection.

12 Remove the needle applying counterpressure with a swab. Gently massage the area over the injection site to aid dispersal of the medicine.

13 Reassure the patient.

14 Remove and dispose of equipment.

15 Record accurately that the medicine has been given.

NOTE. Controlled medicines must also be entered and duly signed in the book kept for this purpose.

Intramuscular injection

Equipment

Syringe 2 to 5 ml

Needles—suggested sizes:

    baby: 25 gauge × 1.6 cm

    older child or very thin adult: 23 gauge × 2.5 cm or 3 cm

    average adult, watery fluids: 21 gauge × 3.8 cm

    average adult, thick fluids: 18 gauge × 3.8 cm

    very obese adult: a longer needle may be required

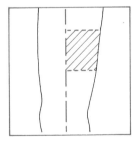 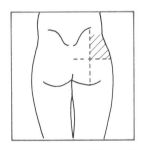

Fig. 14 Sites for intramuscular injection showing (*left*) the mid third of the lateral aspect of the thigh (anterior aspect of left leg illustrated), and (*right*) the upper outer quadrant of the buttock (right buttock shown).

Sites

Anteriolateral aspect of the thigh (quadriceps vastus
    lateralis) (see Fig. 14a).

Anterior part of upper outer quadrant of the but-
    tocks (gluteal muscles) (see Fig. 14b).

Upper outer part of the arm (deltoid muscles).

Giving an intramuscular injection

1   Make skin taut with thumb and forefinger of the
left hand.

2   Hold the syringe like a pan and introduce the
needle smartly at a right angle to the skin (90°).

3   Keep firm counterpressure on the skin with a
swab as the needle is withdrawn.

Hypodermic (subcutaneous) injection

Equipment

Syringe 1 to 2 ml

Needles—suggested sizes:
    baby: 25 gauge × 1.6 cm
    adult: 23 gauge × 2.5 cm

Sites

Fleshy outer part of upper arm.

Fleshy parts of anteriolateral aspects of thigh.

Occasionally anterior abdominal wall, e.g. diabetic
    patients for whom the site must be varied.

Giving a hypodermic injection

1   Take up a small area of tissue between the thumb
and first finger of the left hand.

2   Insert the needle at an angle of 45° (usually in
an upwards direction).

3   Withdraw the piston to ensure the needle has
not entered a blood vessel.

4   Inject the medicine as for intramuscular injection.

Special notes

When a medicine is known to cause sensitivity in staff, disposable gloves and masks should be worn during its preparation and administration, e.g. streptomycin, penicillin, chlorpromazine.

Paraldehyde is administered using a special glass syringe.

Two nurses should help to give an injection to a young child and in other cases when necessary.

When intramuscular injections are repeated frequently, alternate the site of injection.

12.3
Intravenous therapy

Replacement of large amounts of fluid lost from the body, or the correction of serious electrolyte imbalance is more rapidly and accurately dealt with by the introduction of a suitable solution directly into the venous circulation.

There are at least four types of container for intravenous fluids in current use. Each type requires a slight variation in the way it is set up.

Glass bottle
The appropriate needle of the recipient set, after removing its protective sheath, is inserted up to its flange into the rubber bung of the glass bottle.

To minimise coring, the needle must be pushed in by a short stabbing action without twisting and at an angle of 90° to the closure surface (rubber bung).

The air inlet needle is inserted in the same manner, if required, while the bottle is in an upright position and the filter held in such a manner so as to maintain it in a dry condition at the time of suspending.

Polyfusor
Delivery nozzle of the Polyfusor container is cut off with **sterile scissors** and the needle inserted firmly as for the glass bottle. No air inlet is required.

Non-rigid plastic packet
The plastic flaps are pulled apart to reveal the delivery nozzle and the needle of the recipient set inserted firmly as for the glass bottle. No air inlet is required.

Plastic blood pack
The seal from one of the two parts of the blood pack is removed and the needle of the recipient set is inserted by a firm twisting motion. No air inlet is required.

NOTE. Once the uppermost needle of the recipient set has been inserted, fluid is run through the whole of the set to expel air. This is done by allowing the chambers to half fill with fluid and then by releasing the clamp allowing the fluid to run through the entire length of the recipient set. When all the air is expelled, the clamp is closed and the distal end re-covered. The tubing is carefully hung on the drip stand until it can be attached to the cannula.

Equipment
Basic trolley for sterile procedures (see Procedure 3.16) plus on the *Lower shelf* the following additional equipment:
Velcro tourniquet or sphygmomanometer
Arm splint (padded) and bandage
Intravenous cannulae (selection) or as requested by the doctor
Recipient set
Bottle holder (if required)
Prescribed fluid to be administered
Infusion stand taken to the bedside
Shaving equipment for the arm, if necessary

12

If it is necessary to cut down to a vein through the
    tissues, the following items are also required:
2 ml syringe and needles
Local anaesthetic, e.g. lignocaine 1% or 2%
Cut down set containing:
    1 scalpel handle and blade. After use the scalpel
        blade must be disposed of **safely**.
    1 pair of fine toothed dissecting forceps
    1 pair of fine non-toothed dissecting forceps
    1 pair of fine pointed scissors
    2 pairs of straight mosquito forceps
    1 aneurysm needle
    Suturing material
    Intravenous cannula (usually longer than the type
        used for direct venepuncture)

Preparation of the patient
The procedure and reasons for same should be explained to the patient. The patient's arm is shaved,
if required.
    NOTE. If the patient is right-handed the left arm
should be used and vice versa.

Procedure
The procedure is carried out by a doctor assisted by
a nurse.
1   The patient's arm is fully exposed by removing
the sleeve of the gown or pyjama jacket.
2   The doctor cleans the skin area, and the tourniquet or syhygmomanometer cuff is applied (the
latter is inflated) round the upper arm to distend
the distal veins.
3   The doctor inserts the cannula and when blood
appears, the distal end of the recipient tubing is
attached to it and the tourniquet or cuff released
and removed.

4 The flow of the fluid is then adjusted by the clamp of the recipient set and the cannula and tubing are firmly secured to the patient's arm.

5 If splinting is required, the splint should be applied to the patient's arm with a bandage, taking care that it does not impede the flow of the fluid in the vein by external pressure.

6 Make sure that the patient's limb is comfortable and, if necessary, a light covering should be placed over it.

Nursing notes

During the procedure the nurse should observe the patient and attend to his/her comfort and well being. The nurse should also assist the doctor when necessary.

The position of the patient should be as comfortable as possible and the locker must be placed in reach of his/her free arm.

When a splint has been applied, the infusion site should be readily accessible.

The **rate of flow** is maintained according to the doctor's instructions.

Observations

The site of entry of the cannula through the skin should be inspected regularly, i.e. hourly or as instructed, in case the cannula has become dislodged from the vein (see Complications, below)

The patient's pulse rate and temperature are noted and recorded as ordered e.g. $\frac{1}{4}$-1 hourly.

Note should also be made of the patient's colour, any complaints of pain, sweating or other abnormal reactions and the doctor informed.

12

Complications

Any difficulty in maintaining the flow must be reported at once.

Common causes are:

> The top of the cannula may be occluded by the wall of the vein. Slight movement of the limb may correct this.
>
> Spasm of the vein. Gentle stroking of the limb over the vein may help.
>
> Tubing may be kinked or bandage may be too tight.
>
> The cannula may be dislodged and the fluid is infiltrating into the surrounding tissues.
>
> Clot may form in the cannula and block it completely.

Incompatibility of blood may be manifested by pyrexia, rigor, erythema (reddening of the skin) and pain in the lumbar region.

Phlebitis of the vein may cause severe pain and the infusion may have to be stopped and reinserted in another vein.

Sepsis at the cut-down site will be minimised by a high standard of aseptic technique by the operator and those subsequently managing the procedure.

Air embolism is prevented by ensuring that all air is expelled from the tubing of the recipient set.

To change containers

Two nurses, one of whom should be trained, must be present when changing a container.

1   A full container of the correct fluid ordered by the doctor, must be obtained and checked against the written prescription. Check expiry date.

2   When the fluid level is just above the tip of the needle in the container, the clamp should be closed and the container unhooked from the stand. The

apparatus is then transferred to the new container and erected as previously described.

NOTE. All fluids given must be accurately recorded on the patient's IV fluid prescription and fluid balance chart. Record batch number of container on appropriate form.

Discontinuation of infusion or transfusion

When the infusion or transfusion has been discontinued, the apparatus is clamped off, the cannula withdrawn gently and a small sterile dressing applied to the area.

The used apparatus is disposed of carefully with the minimum of handling and the fluid containers or attached labels are returned, if necessary to the appropriate department.

Special note

Intravenous containers **must be carefully inspected prior** to administration. If there is any doubt concerning the contents of the pack **it should not be used**. The pharmacy should be notified and packs of the same batch number should be removed from circulation, pending further instructions.

12.4
Blood transfusion

Crossmatching of blood

1   A specimen (5 ml) of the patient's blood is sent to the blood transfusion centre.

2   The bottle must be accurately and legibly labelled with the full name of the patient, the hospital, the number of the ward, the date of collection and the patient's date of birth.

3   The request form is completed by the doctor. This is a permanent record.

4   It takes $1\frac{1}{2}$ to 2 hours to carry out a full range of grouping and compatibility tests. (The blood specimen, if possible, should be sent to the Blood Transfusion Service 48 hours before the transfusion is to be given.)

5   In an emergency (i.e. clinician decides it is essential to obtain blood for transfusion in less than 2 hours the laboratory will affix a special label to the blood unit stating that it has not been fully crossmatched.

Equipment
As per Procedure 12.3.

Preparation of the patient
As per Procedure 12.3.

Procedure
As per Procedure 12.3 plus the following important additions.

1   Blood collected from blood bank, refrigerator or laboratory by a responsible person. If collected from the refrigerator the following must be recorded on the sheet provided: date, time, patient's name and number of blood pack.

2   Blood **must always be checked** before administration.

(a) Blood checked by a doctor and a nurse or by two nurses, one of whom must be trained.

(b) **Check** particulars on form issued with the blood pack against particulars in the patient's case notes:

    patient's full name
    patient's unit number
    patient's date of birth

(c) **Check** that the blood group and number on the blood pack is the same as that recorded on the form issued with the blood pack.

    NOTE. If (b) and (c) are not all correct notify the Blood Transfusion Service and the doctor. **Do not commence the transfusion.**

    If (b) and (c) are all correct the issued form is signed by two members of the ward staff (see (a)) and attached to the blood pack.

(d) **Check** the patient's identity wristband.

Procedural notes

Normal saline is **always** used before and after a blood transfusion.

Recipient set with a filter and a plastic needle is used for administration of blood. Air inlet is not required.

Blood transfusion must be commenced to run at the correct time and at the correct rate as ordered by the doctor on the patient's IV fluid prescription and fluid balance chart.

12

345

Record number of the blood pack on the patient's
   IV fluid prescription and fluid balance chart.
4 hours should be the maximum time for the administration of one unit (pack) of blood.

Observations
During blood transfusion check the patient's pulse
   rate, temperature and blood pressure are noted
   and recorded as ordered, e.g. $\frac{1}{4}$–1 hourly.
Observe and record the patient's urinary output.
Observe and note the patient's colour, any complaints of pain, sweating, restlessness or other
   abnormal reactions.
If adverse reaction to blood occurs, notify the doctor. If advised, stop the transfusion and the doctor
   will notify the Blood Transfusion Service.
See also Procedure 12.3, Observations.
   NOTE. The pack of blood, with recipient set **still
in situ** is returned to the Blood Transfusion Service.

Incompatibility of blood
An adverse reaction to blood may be manifested by:
   pyrexia
   tachycardia
   rise or fall in blood pressure
   rigor
   erythema
   pain in lumbar region
   jaundice

Complications
See Procedure 12.3.

To change blood containers
As per Procedure 12.3 plus collection and checking
procedures as detailed in this procedure.

Discontinuation of transfusion

As per Procedure 12.3 plus:

1   Form issued with blood pack returned to Blood Transfusion Service.

2   Blood pack placed in disposal bag for disposal in appropriate container.

3   Form giving details of blood transfusion is retained in the patient's case notes.

   NOTE.   Recipient set is changed if an infusion is to continue.

   Normal saline is **always** used before and after a blood transfusion and as directed by medical staff, e.g. between the administration of units of packed cells.

Specific notes

Blood **must always be stored** in designated blood bank refrigerator or refrigerated delivery box.

Blood should not be out of the refrigerator for longer than 30 minutes before administration. It is *dangerous* if frozen. Warm, only if necessary by an approved method. *Danger of overheating* and *contamination* of blood is a serious risk.

If plasma or plasma protein used, a special form is completed and returned to the Blood Transfusion Service.

Dried plasma is reconstituted by mixing it with a special bottle of sterile, distilled water supplied with the dried plasma. The dried plasma should dissolve within 5 minutes—if it does not dissolve or forms gelatinous particles, **do not use**. The dried plasma should be used within 1 hour of being reconstituted.

Warm **fresh frozen plasma** before use (not above 40°C).

For other requests, e.g. Coombs' test, use the designated form. The form is forwarded to the Blood Transfusion Service.

12.5
Moist inhalations

Moist inhalations used in inflammation of the air passages and accessory nasal sinuses to lessen pain and congestion, soothe an irritating cough and loosen secretions.

Equipment
Nelson inhaler
Cork and glass mouthpiece
Cover for the inhaler
Piece of gauze and strapping
Jug of boiling water
Vapourizer if prescribed, e.g. tincture of benzoin or
    menthol crystals
Teaspoon to measure the tincture
Bowl to hold the inhaler
Sputum container

Preparation of equipment
Prepare inhalation.
Cover glass mouthpiece with gauze and secure same
    with strapping.
Fill inhaler with boiling water to just below the level
    of the air inlet, cover and put it in the bowl.

Procedure
1   The covered Nelson inhaler in the bowl is placed in front of the patient on a **firm surface with the air inlet facing away from the patient**.
2   Instruct the patient to place his/her lips on the covered glass mouthpiece and breathe through the mouth and out through the nose.

12

3 The treatment is continued for about 10 minutes.
4 The nurse must stay with elderly patients, children, psychiatric and mentally handicapped patients.
5 The patient should remain in the same atmosphere for 20 minutes after the procedure.

NOTE. If tincture of benzoin is prescribed, 5 ml is added to the boiling water. If menthol crystals are prescribed, one or two crystals are added to the water.

12

12.6
Intravenous therapy in children

See also Procedure 12.3.

Possible sites
1 Superficial vein in hand, foot, arm or leg.
2 Scalp vein.
3 Cut down into deeper veins in the limbs.
4 Long-stay infusion into jugular vein.

Equipment for sites 1 and 2
Basic trolley for sterile procedures (see Procedure 3.16) plus on the *Lower shelf* the following additional equipment:

Velcro tourniquet—nurse can hold arm or leg

Arm splint (correct size for infant or child) and bandage

Intravenous cannulae (selection) or as requested by the doctor

Recipient set with burette incorporated

Bottle holder, if required

Prescribed fluid to be administered

Infusion stand taken to bedside

Infusion pump, if required

Shaving equipment, if necessary

NOTE. Appropriate size elastic band and plaster of Paris strips also required for scalp-vein infusion.

Preparation of the child
A careful explanation of what is to happen **must be given** to the older child and to the parents in the case of infants.

12

If a scalp vein is to be used it will be necessary to shave some hair around the area of the vein selected and the parents should be forewarned of this, if possible.

Procedure

Carried out by a doctor assisted by nurses (see Procedure 12.3).

1   Some restraint is usually necessary and therefore two or three nurses may be required during the procedure for its success.

Older children will require continual reassurance and explanations.

Younger children and babies should be wrapped securely in a blanket with only the desired limb exposed.

2   If a scalp vein is to be used, the baby is wrapped securely in a blanket and placed across the plinth or cot. An elastic band is placed around the baby's head to make the scalp veins stand out. Once the intravenous cannula is in situ the elastic band is carefully cut with round-end scissors. The cannula is anchored with strips of plaster of paris.

3   If arm, hand, foot or leg veins are used, the nurse may be required to hold the limb tightly to make the veins stand out and keep the limb still. Once the intravenous cannula is in situ it is secured with adhesive tape and carefully splinted. (See Nursing notes item 2.)

4   Mitts can be used to prevent toddlers or babies from pulling out or playing with the intravenous cannula or the recipient set.

Equipment for cut down procedure

As previously listed for sites 1 and 2 plus the equipment required for cutting down as per Procedure 12.3.

12

Procedure

1   Procedure carried out by a doctor assisted by a nurse/s.

2   The area of the vein selected is prepared observing strict asepsis.

3   A local anaesthetic may be administered.

4   An incision is made and the selected deep vein is exposed. The cannula is inserted and the incision is then sutured to keep the cannula in position.

5   The limb is then carefully splinted.

NOTE. **Long-stay infusion into jugular vein** is usually undertaken under theatre conditions. The patient is anaesthetised or heavily sedated.

Types of intravenous fluids used in paediatric nursing

Sodium chloride 0.18% and dextrose 4% (most widely used intravenous fluid in paediatric nursing)

Sodium chloride 0.45% and dextrose 5%

Sodium chloride 0.9%

Dextrose 5%

Hartmann's solution

Changing containers

As per Procedure 12.3.

Observations

As per Procedure 12.3 plus regular and frequent checks on the infusion site especially a scalp vein infusion.

Nursing notes

1   Fluid balance is of **paramount importance** in children. There is a far greater risk, than with an adult patient, of overloading the circulatory system with the possibility of ensuing cardiac failure.

The 24-hour total of fluid to be administered is calculated by the clinician in charge and written instructions signed by a doctor as to the rate of flow in millilitres per hour are given to the nursing staff. These instructions **are strictly adhered to**. Allowing intravenous fluid to infuse either too quickly or too slowly in 1 hour and balancing it over the next hour **is not acceptable** and indeed might have serious consequences.

The paediatric IV fluid prescription and fluid balance chart allows for accurate assessment of all types of fluid intake and output on an hourly basis.

24-hour fluid balance is calculated at a suitably designated time, e.g. 8.00 a.m. or 8.00 p.m.

The number of the bottle or container in the sequence and the batch number must be recorded on the IV fluid prescription and fluid balance chart.

In small infants and children a recipient set calibrated to give 60 drops in every millilitre of intravenous fluid used.

2   Satisfactory splintage is of **paramount importance** to maintain the intravenous cannula in position. It is sometimes possible, in dealing with scalp-vein infusions to limit head movement with the use of sand bags but it **must be remembered** that scalp veins are friable and puncture easily and therefore depending on the situation it may be necessary for sedation to be prescribed for the baby.

3   The setting up of an intravenous infusion can sometimes be very difficult and at best is a traumatic experience for any child. Therefore, nurses **must be extremely vigilant** in their observations and nursing care to ensure that the intravenous cannula remains in situ and that the fluid absorbed as per the written instructions.

4   If there is a choice in the site of the intravenous

12

infusion, the doctor might be asked to leave the thumbsucking or writing hand of the child free.

Intravenous pump
If an intravenous pump is in use nurses must be alert to the alarm going off. If the pump alarms repeatedly carry out the following:
    check the position of the electronic eye and tubing
    check the position of the limb
    inspect the site of the infusion
If the alarm continues inform the doctor.

Complications
As per Procedure 12.3.

Discontinuation of infusion
As per Procedure 12.3.

12.7
Administration of oral medicines to children

While administering medicine to children, all the cardinal rules apply but are **even more important**. Errors if they do occur have a far greater impact, indeed some may be irreversible or even fatal.

Medicine dosage is calculated on a *weight basis* and consequently different fractions of the adult dose will result for each individual child. This requires the nurse to be able to calculate the dose ordered from the stock dose and she/he must be able to show how the answer is reached.

It also means that every child's weight **must be displayed** clearly at the top of the medicine kardex so that it is readily available when the doctor prescribes for the child. The admission weight is usually charted and if the child requires treatment over a long period or, if there is considerable change in the child's weight pattern, the medicine kardex is amended as required.

See also Procedure 12.1.

Rules for medicine administration in children

All medicine **must be** ordered and signed for by a doctor on the child's medicine prescription sheet.

No verbal instruction should be taken over the telephone unless in a dire emergency.

There **must be two nurses** administering medicines, one of whom must be trained.

12

Two nurses are necessary for checking purposes and to assist with administration of medicines to small children.

Careful signing of medicines given is required by both nurses.

The medicine trolley must accompany the nurses on the medicine round and **must never** be left unattended. **Always** lock the trolley if called away in an emergency.

The medicine keys should remain on the person of the nurse in charge of the ward or the senior nurse administering the medicines in order to minimise the number of persons handling the keys. The key **should never be** given to junior members of staff.

Identify the name of the patient with the name on the medicine prescription sheet and the child's identity wristband.

Check medicine sensitivity column.

Read the prescription carefully.

Select the medicine and check the label with the prescription. Shake all medicines well, particularly antibiotics in suspension. Ensure that the label is kept clean (if liquid medicine) by holding the bottle with label uppermost against the palm of the pouring hand.

Hold the medicine glass at eye level while pouring the medicine.

All medicines given in liquid form **must be measured** in a glass measure, or a syringe, if the dosage is very small and **transferred to a plastic or polythene measure or spoon** for administration. **Never give a glass measure to a child**—he/she may bite through the glass and cause injury.

If a medicine is in suspension or syrup form **always**

check the expiry date as suspensions activated by the addition of water last in their active state for only 7 days. The date of dispensing or activation needs to be written on the bottle label.

When administering powders, place in a plastic or polythene measure and mix well with a small amount of diluted fruit juice.

Administer teeth staining medicines with a straw.

Administer effervescent tablets with diluted fruit juice.

Make unpleasant medicines as agreeable as possible by following their administration with a drink of juice. Sometimes it is possible to mix powders with a spoonful of jam. **Never mix medicines with milk or add to a baby's feed.** You may give the child a dislike of milk or if he/she does not finish the feed he/she will not have taken all of the medicine prescribed.

Small children and babies should wear bibs to prevent spillage on to their clothes.

There are many ways of persuading children to take medicines but as the medicine therapy will be an important part of the child's treatment there is no question about it, the child must be persuaded to take the medicine. If children are approached in a matter of fact way with their medicine, they will usually accept it.

It is important **never** to leave a child's medicine on the locker and it is necessary to stay with the child until the medicine is swallowed.

Any difficulties noted on the medicine round **must be reported** to the nurse in charge, e.g. medicines which have been vomited. It is then the responsibility of the nurse in charge to contact the doctor with regard to repeating the dose. **This must never be done without medical advice.**

12

12.8
Administration of medicines in the community

NOTE. All medicines are the property of the patient.

Oral medicines
The district nursing sister/charge nurse has the responsibility to supervise and advise any patient she/he may be visiting who is taking oral medicines and to report back to the general practitioner.

Medicines by injection
Any medicine administered by injection **must be** carefully checked, recorded and signed for. The name of the nurse administering the medicine **must be** written in full. Initials must never be used.

Immunisation
Immunisation must only be undertaken in accordance with local policy.

Controlled medicines
All controlled medicines **must be administered** by a registered nurse.

Written and signed instructions from the general practitioner **must be kept** in the patient's home.

The prescription and the dosage must be carefully read and checked.

Whenever possible a suitable responsible relative should be trained to double check.

Medicine, dose administered, time given and amount of medicine left must be recorded and signed for in the record sheet left in the patient's home.

When controlled medicines are discontinued, it is the responsibility of the district nursing sister/charge nurse to ensure, with the relative's consent that such medicines are destroyed. The relative should destroy the medicine supervised and witnessed by the district nursing sister/charge nurse. A note to this effect signed by the relative and the nurse should be attached to the patient's record card.

If such medicines are not destroyed, it is the duty of the district nursing sister/charge nurse to inform the general practitioner of this. The nurse should note on the patient's record card the medicine, amount left in the patient's home and that she/he has notified the general practitioner.

In certain cases the district nursing sister/charge nurse may wish to discuss with the general practitioner the refusal of the relative to destroy the medicine.

Insulin

All requirements for administration of insulin should be kept together in a suitable container and all patients should have a spare syringe.

Each patient must have a specially prepared **diabetic notebook.** The following information must be detailed on the inside front cover:

the patient's name and address
the district nursing sister's/charge nurse's name
the patient's general practitioner's name and telephone number

The dosage, type and strength of the insulin

12

prescribed **must be clearly written** at the top of each page.

When there is a change in the dosage, type of strength of the insulin prescribed, the page containing the **former insulin prescription must be scored through with one diagonal line marked (dosage changed)** and the **new insulin prescribed clearly written on a new page.**

Extreme caution must be observed when checking and re-checking each patient's administration of insulin. The following procedure must be followed:

1   Ascertain the dose, type and strength from the patient's diabetic notebook.

2   Check the insulin for type, strength and expiry date. Check type and strength with the **current** insulin prescription.

3   Draw up the amount of insulin to be administered.

4   Re-check that the correct amount has been drawn up according to the strength of the insulin.

5   After administration of the insulin, enter date, time and dosage in the patient's diabetic notebook and **sign** against the entry.

6   The dosage **must be** recorded in **units**.

The patient's diabetic notebook should accompany him/her when he/she has an appointment at the diabetic out-patient clinic.

Index

Index

Index

Index

Index